A Refuge of Cure or Care

A Refuge of Cure or Care

The Sensory Dimensions of Confinement at the Worcester State Hospital for the Insane

Madeline Kearin Ryan

LEXINGTON BOOKS
Lanham • Boulder • New York • London

Published by Lexington Books
An imprint of The Rowman & Littlefield Publishing Group, Inc.
4501 Forbes Boulevard, Suite 200, Lanham, Maryland 20706
www.rowman.com

6 Tinworth Street, London SE11 5AL, United Kingdom

British Library Cataloguing in Publication Information Available

Library of Congress Cataloging-in-Publication Data Available

ISBN 978-1-7936-4381-0 (cloth)
ISBN 978-1-7936-4383-4 (pbk)
ISBN 978-1-7936-4382-7 (electronic)

Contents

Introduction   1

1   "Curious Relics" and "Drafty Corridors": The Material
World of the Asylum   35

2   "A State of Conscious and Permanent Visibility": Sight as an
Instrument of Cure and Control   69

3   "As Syllable from Sound": The Sonic Dimensions of
Confinement   103

4   The Smell of the Insane: Disciplining the Olfactory Domain   129

5   Dirty Bread, Forced Feeding, and Tea Parties:
The Uses and Abuses of Food   155

Discussion: The Disorderly Sensorium   187

Conclusion: The Afterlife of the Asylum   201

Bibliography   205

Index   223

About the Author   227

Introduction

Insane asylums are frequently depicted as haunted relics of a time when mentally ill people were imprisoned and abused. Yet at the time the first American state hospitals were built in the early nineteenth century, the asylum was conceptualized neither as an instrument for controlling the deviant nor as "a dumping ground for society's disaffected" (Beveridge 1997), but as a "technological marvel" that would solve the country's mental health crisis and alleviate the suffering of thousands (Yanni 2007). The asylum was viewed as a "panacea equivalent to the steam engine, the rights of man, or the spread of universal knowledge" (Bynum and Shepherd 1985: 3); like the visions of Arcadia conjured by contemporary utopian communities, it offered a solution to the dislocations and ruptures of modernity. The crumbling clock towers and gutted wards that today constitute the ruined asylum landscape "were once monuments to civic pride, built with noble intentions by leading architects and physicians who envisioned asylums as places of refuge, therapy, and healing" (Payne 2009: 13).

In order to understand the promise these institutions once embodied in the public imagination and how that promise ultimately soured, it is necessary to articulate the mechanics through which asylums were intended to function as therapeutic instruments. Their curative architecture was predicated on three core beliefs. The first was that insanity was a "disease of civilization" (Grob 1966; Murat 2014) to be conceptualized—and treated—foremost in environmental terms. The second was that insanity was curable, and could be remedied by the patient's removal to a quiet, isolated, pastoral setting in which daily life was organized according to "natural" laws (Browne 1837; Scull 1981). The third was the conviction that physicians and architects, in partnership, were uniquely positioned to solve the "insanity problem"

1

(Yanni 2007). Physicians' faith in these tenets, and the willingness of state and private benefactors to underwrite their ameliorative efforts in the name of the public good, fueled the construction and expansion of state hospitals throughout the United States, beginning in the early nineteenth century and peaking in 1960, when they collectively housed more than half a million people (Markowitz 2006).

As one of the first state hospitals in the United States, the Worcester State Hospital in Worcester, Massachusetts, set a precedent that would be replicated across the country (Grob 1966). Because the senses were believed to provide a direct conduit into a person's mental condition, the curative force of the Worcester State Hospital was thought to reside in its command over sensory experience. Its extensive lawn and grounds provided access to nature unspoiled by the pollution and noise of urban life. The chapel provided a setting for the enjoyment of sacred music and exposure to positive moral influence that functioned as a counterweight to modern vices and dissipation. Patients were served a wholesome diet with food supplied from the asylum farm: the literal fruits of their own labor. The founders of the Worcester State Hospital hoped that the institution would provide "this unfortunate class of our fellow beings" with "every benefit which can be derived from a favorable change in their physical sensations, combined with a change of residence, of regiment [*sic*], and of moral treatment" (Trustees 1832: 32).

In the following pages, I discuss how the particular configurations of sight, sound, touch, smell, and taste produced by the Worcester State Hospital were mobilized in the moral architecture of its therapeutic environment. I compare the ambitious theory underlying the design of the asylum with its often messy realization in the face of chronic overcrowding and underfunding, and describe how this disjuncture shaped the texture of patient experiences. In doing so, I attempt to reconstruct "the contingent co-presence of heterogeneous elements such as bodies, things, substances, affects, memories, information, and ideas" that constituted the Worcester State Hospital: what Yannis Hamilakis terms a "sensorial assemblage" (Hamilakis 2014: 126). This concept forms a node in the juncture between the fields of medical anthropology, phenomenology, and the historical archaeology of institutions, all of which build from the premise that the environment does not simply represent a stage for action, but acts as a vessel, instrument, and creator of meaning. Accordingly, by reconstructing the sensorial assemblage of the Worcester State Hospital, I argue, it is possible to distinguish the role of the five senses in framing the conception and lived experience of insanity in the nineteenth century, including the ways in which individual agency articulates with and against the sensory configurations of the asylum.

THE BIRTH OF THE ASYLUM

The "belief in the power of carefully designed institutions to effect social change" was a phenomenon unique to the nineteenth century (Tomes 1984: 131). Prior to the emergence of this belief, so-called lunatics were generally maintained in their native communities. Those for whom medical treatment was accessible and affordable might be treated in their homes by a physician using a limited arsenal of remedies, including bleeding and purging; alternately, they might receive the ministrations of a cleric who sought to absolve them of the sins that were thought to have contributed to their condition. Lunatics without resources were supported by "outdoor" relief (as opposed to "indoor," institutional care) in the form of benefits paid to the family supporting them. These "non-institutional mechanisms" for "treating both the dependent and the delinquent" were adapted to the relatively small agrarian communities of colonial America, which were bound together by informal ties of mutual obligation (Rothman 2002: 160). The burgeoning of industrial capitalism and the resulting growth and mobility of the population frayed these social bonds. Geographic isolation and lack of job security further deprived workers of their traditional support networks.

By the late eighteenth and early nineteenth centuries, members of the upper and middle classes were becoming acutely aware of the dissonance between the newly elaborated republican ideal of social equality and the crushing realities of poverty, disease, and crime. In contrast to previous generations, who viewed the existence of paupers, lunatics, and other aberrant figures as part of the natural fabric of society, the new mercantile bourgeoisie believed that deviance presented a problem that demanded a solution. Highly educated, deeply spiritual, and aspiring toward gentility, members of this class possessed an unprecedented faith in human progress (Tomes 1984: 39; Bushman 2003). Their faith was underwritten by the religious currents of the Second Great Awakening that portrayed mankind as advancing rapidly toward a perfected state culminating in the new millennium (Grob 1966: 45). Industrial technologies and the capital furnished by the market economy offered the tools necessary to realize their goals. The total institution was the product of this synthesis. Within the institution, the body of the inmate acted as a metonym for society, through which administrators sought to cure what was pathological in the new social order (Altschuler 2018: 29). Almshouses, workhouses, prisons, and boarding schools each targeted a particular locus of disease with the aim of rendering a healthy body politic.

Like other total institutions, the drive underlying the creation of asylums for the insane was couched foremost in humanitarian terms. The lunatic hospital formed the center of a new approach to madness known as moral treatment, which was first elaborated in France and England in the late eighteenth century and subsequently imported into the United States. Departing from earlier beliefs that lunatics were flawed beyond the hope of redemption, moral treatment emphasized their humanity. The English branch of moral treatment represented an elaboration of the religious principles of the Society of Friends or Quakers, which called for "the law of love and sympathy," in contrast to the harsh confinement and heroic medical measures of earlier generations (Annual Report 1834: 6; Cherry 1989, Gamwell and Tomes 1984). The proponents of moral treatment emphasized "careful attention to cleanliness, exercise, air, and substantial diet" as a means of supporting the total health of the patient (Annual Report 1833: 6). The belief that insanity was essentially the result of an unbalanced physiology justified the conviction that a return to moderate habits would reliably effect a cure in all but the most severe cases (Coventry 1846).

The insane asylum formed part of a larger movement in the nineteenth century that enshrined a particular vision of preindustrial Nature as a panacea to the ills of industrialization. This nostalgia for the past sought to recover the experiences, landscapes, and values that were believed to be under threat by the forces of modernity. Rural cemeteries, public parks, private gardens, and the artistic works produced by the Hudson River School of painting all represented expressions of this impulse to stall the effects of time. The "taste for an idealized Nature had revolutionary implications," leading to a new orientation toward the built environment and the growth of a "picturesque aesthetic" that "compos[ed] natural and manmade features into harmonious wholes" (Bushman 1993: 245; Linden 1989: 29). Designed in accordance with a Romantic view of nature, the asylum offered a refuge from the pathological scenes of modern civilization (Grob 1966: 57). Like the paradisiacal community described in Elihu Hubbard Smith's "The Institutions of the Republic of Utopia," asylum architects envisioned a "salubrious closed system" in which "healthy land makes citizens healthy" and "labor ensures the health of their bodies, the land, and the republic" (Altschuler 2016: 37). The hospital was not simply a site for moral treatment, but its most important instrument. Invigorated by the reported successes of their peers in Europe, American physicians were incredibly optimistic, projecting a cure rate of 90% for patients who were treated promptly in an asylum. Their vision formed the model for the Worcester State Hospital and its successors. However, asylum administrators would soon realize the difficulty of creating an ideal environment, and of marshaling the financial and human capital necessary to sustain it. The arc of asylum history closely shadows that experienced by many utopian communities: beginning with a swell of enthusiasm; followed by the systematic erosion of its early successes by bureaucratic entanglements, lack of resources, and the vagaries of human behavior; and ending in disappointment and disillusionment.

DEFINING INSANITY

The medical definition of insanity over the course of the nineteenth century represented an ongoing negotiation between materialist and spiritualist doctrines. While physicians recognized the mind and the body as distinct entities, they posited the existence of a mechanism for sympathetic communication between the two that was capable of translating moral and emotional disturbance into physical disorder and, in turn, translating physical disorder into insanity (Cox 1811: 57). Experiences such as "disappointed ambition" and behaviors such as masturbation and intemperance did not *directly* drive a person insane, but rather created the conditions for insanity to develop by disturbing the brain. The focus on the brain as the locus for insanity was crucial to physicians' project to legitimize insanity as a *medical* disease. In objectifying and materializing insanity, physicians were able to secure a monopoly over its management, edging out the religious clerics who had once been their chief competitors (Scull 1979: 159). Yet at the same time, physicians were careful to avoid charges of atheism by upholding the idea of a spiritual essence that remained intact in spite of bodily disorder. Insanity could not touch the true seat of the soul: "the mind, [even] in the most deplorable case, is not obliterated," but merely "disturbed" (Morris 1851: 18).

The medical claim to insanity was further bolstered by physicians' promises of cure. As soon as the pernicious influences acting upon the brain were removed, "a healthy condition of the brain [would be] restored," and "reason again resumes its empire" (Annual Report 1839: 65). Cures for insanity depended on returning the body and mind to a state of equilibrium, which could only be achieved through a healthy environment. The asylum should mimic the "moral order of the family" (Tomes 1984: 42), with a superintendent who acted as a paternal figure and attendants to supervise patients' "conduct, manners, language, dress, appearance, food, exercise, occupations, [and] amusements" (Conolly 1847: 110). Physicians used the asylum as a scaffold through which to reinvent existing moral and religious precepts as the laws of nature. This "tendency to conflate social and scientific truths" was based on the "assumption of unity between natural and divine law" (Tomes 1984: 87). The "natural" laws articulated and enforced by physicians existed in explicit opposition to the "artificial" conditions of modern life that were thought to have contributed to an apparent rise of insanity in the nineteenth century. Artifice and nature, disease and health, vice and morality were juxtaposed within the dichotomous philosophy of moral treatment. According to this scheme, the mechanisms underlying insanity were not shrouded in mystery, but were explicable by common-sense logic. In the words of Dr. Samuel B. Woodward, the first superintendent of the Worcester State Hospital, "insanity is a calculable agency":

We see why it befalls and how it may be averted. We see, that should we all obey certain laws, which are annexed to our being, and are the conditions of enjoying mental soundness, we should be exempt from its power; but we also see, that if we will transgress rules, to whose violation the dreadful consequences of insanity have been attached, it is as certain as to befall us, as fire is to burn. (Annual Report 1838: 6)

The leading causes for insanity listed for the patients of the Worcester State Hospital in 1838, ranked in order of frequency, were "intemperance," "ill health of all kinds," "masturbation," "domestic afflictions," "religious excitements," "loss of property and fear of poverty," "disappointed ambition," "injuries to the head," and "use of snuff/tobacco" (Annual Report 1838: 7). This list helps to explain why insanity was viewed as a "disease of civilization": many of these causes could be traced to new social and economic trends that transformed traditional concepts of family, productivity, and respectability. On an individual basis, the constant threat of destitution caused by the uncertain job market might elicit a level of distress that was capable of inciting mental disorder. To take a more expansive view, the anxieties of the individual worker stood for the anxieties of society as a whole, betraying an ambivalence toward industrialization as a source of both prosperity and poverty, progress and dissipation.

THE ROLE OF THE SENSES IN THE NINETEENTH-CENTURY ASYLUM

The centrality of the senses in the therapeutic paradigms underlying the nineteenth-century asylum derived partly from the writings of John Locke, who posited that "all ideas come from sensation and reflection" and "all knowledge is founded on experience" (Locke 1853: 75). Building on this model of human understanding, the founders of moral treatment theorized that the senses represented both the point of origin for insanity and the proper target for its cure. Their efforts to create the ideal asylum represented a microcosm of the larger project of Western modernity to exert "order, predictability, [and] control" over the realm of the senses as a means of shaping and controlling knowledge (Bauman 1993: 24). Sensory experience played a multifaceted and expanding role in the emergent biomedical paradigm. The sensorium of the physician was enlisted as an instrument of "medical semiology," allowing for accurate diagnosis through "medical observation . . . of the organs and their modifiers, [which] can be pursued only by means of the senses" (Corbin 1986: 40, Broussais 1831: 277). At the same time, the sensory perceptions of the patient became the focus of both etiology and treatment.

The medicalization of insanity depended on a theory of "reciprocal action" between body and mind, as mediated by the senses. In *An Inquiry into the Nature and Origin of Mental Derangement* (1798), Alexander Crichton attributed "erroneous mental perception"—that is, the delusions of insanity—to "diseases of the external senses," stating that "phrenzy" often manifested first as "a disordered state of sensorial feeling" (Crichton 1798: 167). Because mental disorder was attributed to pathological sensory perceptions, physicians theorized that "it may be possible to put the [insane] man's thoughts in the usual and normal course by impressions to be made on his senses" (Broussais 1831: 277). Joseph Mason Cox, in *Practical Observations on Insanity,* suggested that the insane might find "relief . . . through the medium of the senses," including "music," "placing the patient in an airy room," "flowers," and green-painted "walls and furnitures" (Cox 1811: 101). These theories were embedded in the philosophical structure of the Worcester State Hospital and gained widespread circulation through Woodward's annual reports, in which he wrote that insanity was the result of the "false impressions conveyed to the mind" by the senses, and could be relieved by restoring "a healthy condition of the brain" by means of sensory influence (Annual Report 1839: 65).

Psychiatry continued to depend on the Lockean model of the interaction between mind, body, and senses throughout the nineteenth century. Writing in the *American Journal of Insanity* in 1874, Dr. C. H. Hughes couched Locke's theory in the evolving language of biomedicine, stating that "every manifest *phenomenon* of mind is the result or accompaniment to our senses of some change molecular, chemical or vital in the nervous elements of the brain," and postulating that scientists "may someday find those atomic changes [that] *accompany, precede,* and *follow* the rational and irrational manifestations of mind" (Hughes 1874: 33, 36–37). While this statement suggested that psychiatrists were growing ever closer to discovering the microscopic mechanics underlying mental pathology, the cure for that pathology remained largely the same as it had been at the start of the century. The asylum retained its primacy because it allowed psychiatrists to control the "stimuli addressing the senses," including "all external circumstances and conditions in the situations, surroundings, and relations of the patient, which may have an influence upon states of mind or feeling" (Bancroft 1889: 374). Psychiatrists continued to experiment with "adjustments" to the sensory environment of the asylum into the 1890s, exploring "the instrumentality of the skin," "electricity," "the salutary influence of heat and cold, the sense of smell by means of ethereal substances," and "self-medication through colored glass" (Blumer 1892: 350).

Patients also acknowledged the centrality of the senses in shaping their experiences of the asylum. Clifford Beers, a Yale graduate who was confined to a series of Connecticut asylums between 1900 and 1905, wrote that during the acute phase of his mental illness "*all* of my senses became perverted": "The tricks played upon me by my senses of taste, touch, smell, and sight were the source of great mental anguish" (Beers 1913: 15). Unfortunately, the abuse and neglect he suffered in the course of his commitment served to compound, rather than alleviate, this painfully heightened sensibility. Even those patients who did not consider themselves insane articulated their experiences of confinement largely through the medium of sensory perception. The distinctive and inescapable aurality of the asylum, for example, was a source of distress to many patients and a reoccurring feature of their accounts. Ebenezer Haskell, a mechanic who was committed to the Pennsylvania Hospital for the Insane in 1868, complained of the "violent patients" who "howled and made a great noise all night, around me" (Haskell 1868: 14). At the Troy Lunatic Asylum in New York in the 1870s, Moses Swan spent "many sleepless nights, listening to the screeches and yells of the inmates" (Swan 1874: 47). Upon her commitment to the Worcester State Hospital in 1878, schoolteacher Elizabeth R. Hill "begged" her attendants "to give me a room where I might not hear the talk or see the insane," yet was forced to contend with "the most loathsome, incoherent yells and shrieks that could be made by the most raven lost minds" (Hill 1881: 34).

These accounts suggest that patients shared their physicians' belief in the power of the senses to constitute experience and shape the mind. However, the "sensorial assemblage" rendered collectively in their writings is one that is decidedly pathological, rather than therapeutic, in nature. A central theme, reiterated through almost every patient account, is that of the horrifying irony of an asylum that is capable of *causing* insanity in a sane person. Haskell wrote that the "treatment" dispensed at the Pennsylvania Hospital—where "insane men and women [were] confined to the floor" in "badly constructed and worse ventilated cells"—"would drive a sane man mad"[1] (Haskell 1868: 50). Nellie Bly, an investigative journalist who was shocked by the abuse of patients she witnessed while undercover at the Blackwell's Island Asylum in New York City, posed the question in her groundbreaking exposé: "What, excepting torture, would produce insanity quicker than this treatment?" (Bly 1887). Although Isaac Hunt acknowledged that he was "a wild maniac" when he was committed to the Maine State Hospital in 1851, he believed that "under humane treatment, I should have recovered"; instead, his tortuous experiences in the asylum threw him into a deep depression (Hunt 1851: 3).

Robert Fuller and Elizabeth Packard, both of whom likened their confinement to the Spanish Inquisition, contrasted the humanitarian promise of the lunatic hospital against its shocking realities. Describing the McLean Asylum, to which he was committed in 1832, Fuller wrote that "instead of happiness, it gives distress: instead of health, sickness: instead of life, death: and instead of being an instrument of benevolence, it is made an instrument of extortion" (Fuller 1833: 28). Packard, who successfully sued for her release from the Jacksonville Asylum in the Illinois State Supreme Court in 1862, directed her condemnation at the physician-superintendent, Dr. Andrew McFarland:

> Your discipline is invariably calculated to increase [patients'] difficulties, and make them worse rather than better. Even a person with a sound mind, and a sound body, could hardly pass through a course here and come out unharmed, without faith. A person is very apt to *become* what they are taken to *be*. (Packard 1873: 120–121)

Not much effort is needed to locate "the gap between the rhetoric and the reality of the built environment and life within it for the inmate" of an asylum (Piddock 2007: 219); patients were well aware of this divergence, and articulated it minutely in their accounts. Their explicit descriptions of asylum life, unvarnished by the idealism of physicians and administrators, present a challenge and a provocation to the benevolent reputation of the asylum—but not to its underlying premise.

As Packard wrote, "what the people have regarded as noble institutions of charity, have [become] foul prisons, where savage discipline has taken the place of kind, curative treatment" (Packard 1873: 400). Journalist Albert Deutsch, describing the state hospital system in 1946, made a similar observation, writing that "a potentially powerful organ for betterment [has been] transformed into what was, an effect, a cloak for evil and abuses" (Deutsch 1948: 169). These statements suggest that the failures of moral treatment are attributable not to its theoretical framework, but rather to its faulty execution. Neither physicians nor patients challenged the therapeutic potential of asylums; yet this potential was discarded through the process of deinstitutionalization. Once tarnished by the stain of neglect, abuse, and bureaucratic waste, the asylum was condemned as irredeemable. In this book, I do not attempt to render a judgment on the overall character, success or failure of the asylum. Instead, I advance the senses as a heuristic device for organizing the heterogeneity of experiences encompassed by the asylum, and for understanding how this heterogeneity constituted an institution that could be *both* therapeutic and pathological, curative and custodial, all at once and at different times and places throughout its history.

THE WORCESTER STATE HOSPITAL: A BRIEF HISTORY

In 1829, the Massachusetts legislature ordered the formation of a committee to investigate the condition of its insane citizens in every municipality in the state. The investigation uncovered deplorable scenes of lunatics "dressed in rags" in "dark dungeons," with "no bed, filthy straw, no orifice for light, [and] air so fetid as to produce nauseousness" (The Committee 1830: 20). The committee concluded that under these circumstances, "any improvement of their minds could hardly be expected": a statement that speaks to the ascendance of the new moral treatment paradigm. A few decades earlier, few would have believed that "improvement" of lunatics was possible, much less that it could be effected through a change of scenery, good habits, and kindness. Furthermore, the state would not have made such a claim to responsibility over the welfare of lunatics, which was thought to rightfully belong to their respective communities.[2]

The resolve passed by the state legislature on March 10, 1830, to erect a lunatic hospital with a capacity for 120 patients thus signals a major transformation in views surrounding insanity and the role of the state in managing public welfare. Legislators couched their decision in pragmatic terms, stating that the asylum would "restore" lunatics to a condition of health that would relieve their "burden upon the State" (The Committee 1837: 20). This declaration suggests that the state's action was predicated upon a contractual formulation of citizenship that linked public health to productivity. A healthy body politic was composed of workers who justified their existence on the basis of their economic contribution.

A "pioneer state in the establishment of a central public welfare body," Massachusetts was already distinguished as the site of the first general hospital (Deutsch 1946: 248). The factors underlying the creation of Massachusetts General in 1811—including "the wealth of a rising merchant class, a heightened sense of social obligation, and the determination to achieve complete respectability" (Eaton 1957: 27)—were the same that drove the establishment of the lunatic hospital. Viewed as a progressive and humanitarian institution, the asylum was intended to enshrine the ideals of its founders in material form. Legislators, philanthropists, and physicians were eager to erect what they believed would be "a noble monument of the munificence and public spirit of the state" (Annual Report 1837: 71).

The commissioners tasked with the planning of the hospital initially vacillated between Worcester and Boston, ultimately settling upon the former for its more central location in the state (Grob 1966: 31). While Worcester had yet to ascend to the social and economic stature it would achieve at mid-century, it was poised to become an important hub in developing trade networks, as well as a center for intellectual and reform activity (Eaton 1957: 229). Members of the local mercantile elite were eager to claim the hospital for Worcester as a means of drawing "state patronage" and prestige to the up-and-coming town, and contributed to its development by serving on its board of trustees and purchasing bonds to underwrite its construction (ibid.).

Under the principles of the new curative paradigm, the siting of the asylum itself was thought to play a crucial role in shaping its therapeutic environment. Accordingly, the commissioners were purposeful in their choice of location, selecting a 12-acre plot on Summer Street (figure 0.1) on the outskirts of Worcester that they described as

> a singularly regular and beautiful elevation, commanding a view of the town, and the rich scenery of the surrounding country, sufficiently near to the market, and principal places of business for necessary accommodation, yet so retired as to be secured from improper intrusion or disturbance, and within a short distance of the head waters of the Blackstone Canal. (The Committee 1837: 6)

The next consideration was the building itself. Moral treatment called for "an edifice" that was "materially different, both in form and in interior arrangement, from ordinary habitations" (The Committee 1830). Commissioners needed to meet the basic needs for warmth, light, and fresh air, and to provide a reasonable degree of comfort while also securing the building against patients' potential violence and escape. Because moral treatment stressed the importance of classification, the building would require sufficient accommodations to allow for the segregation of patients into separate wards. Additionally, the building needed to convey the nobility of its enterprise, ensuring that it would bring pride to its current and potential benefactors. In order to achieve these multiple and sometimes conflicting aims, the commissioners turned to an emergent genre of guidebooks that formalized the principles for building an insane asylum. Samuel Tuke's *Practical Hints on the Construction and Economy of Pauper Lunatic Asylums* (1815) was most likely among the sources consulted by the commissioners, as they chose to incorporate a window design identical to that used at Tuke's York Retreat (Tuke 1815: 40).[3]

The layout of the Worcester State Hospital also adhered to Tuke's suggestions, comprising two symmetric wings—one for men and one for women—branching from a central administration building that would house the superintendent, his family, and other employees (figure 0.2). Patients in each wing would be further segregated based on their social standing and type of illness. The building's Neo-Palladian facade echoed that of the private McLean Asylum in Boston, a country mansion that had been retrofitted for hospital use in 1811 by its original architect, Charles Bulfinch (Little 1972: 15). Unlike McLean, the Worcester State Hospital was built with a close attention to expenses, utilizing brick instead of the more expensive granite (The Committee 1830). With the addition of gardens for recreation and fields for agricultural employment, the hospital was fully equipped to meet the standards for moral treatment, with one important exception: the superintendent.

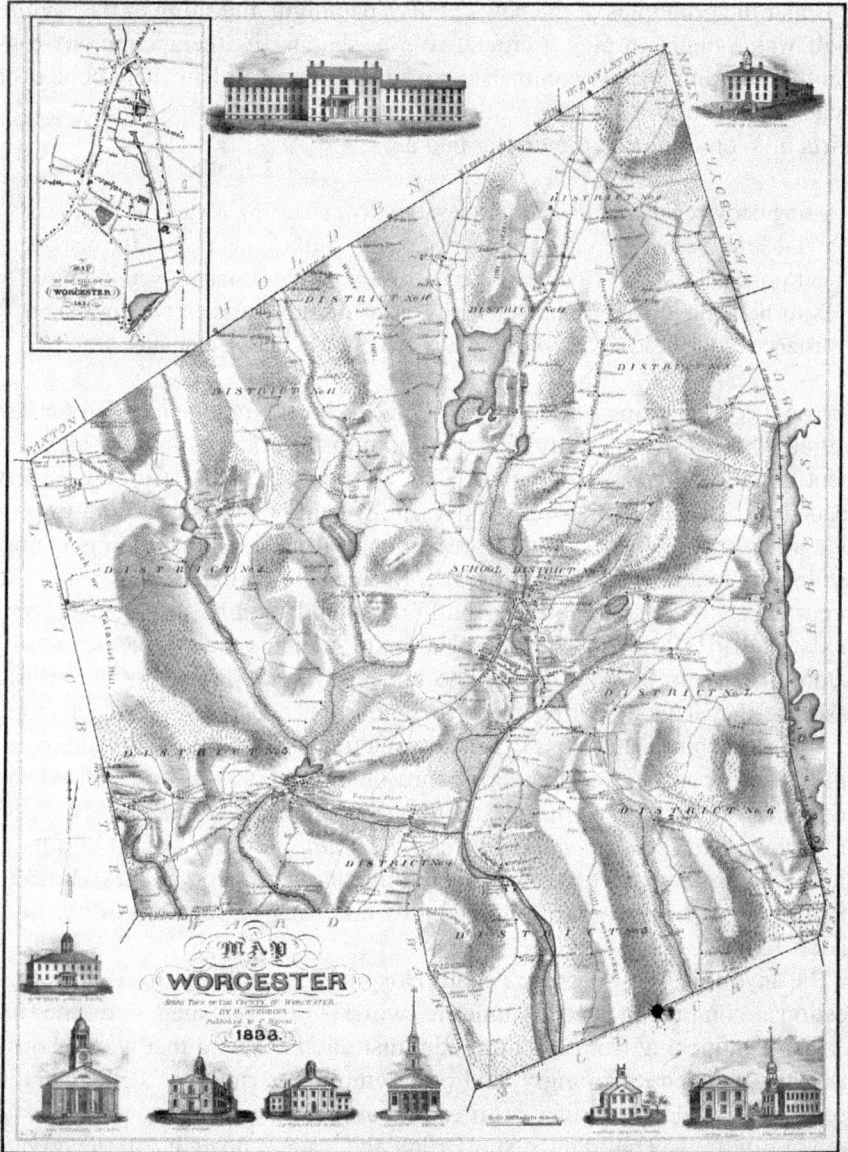

Figure 0.1   Detail of an 1833 Map Showing the Location of the First Worcester State Hospital on Summer Street. Heman Stebbins, A map of Worcester: Shire town of the county of Worcester. C. Harris, Worcester, Mass., 1831. Courtesy of the Harvard Map Collection.

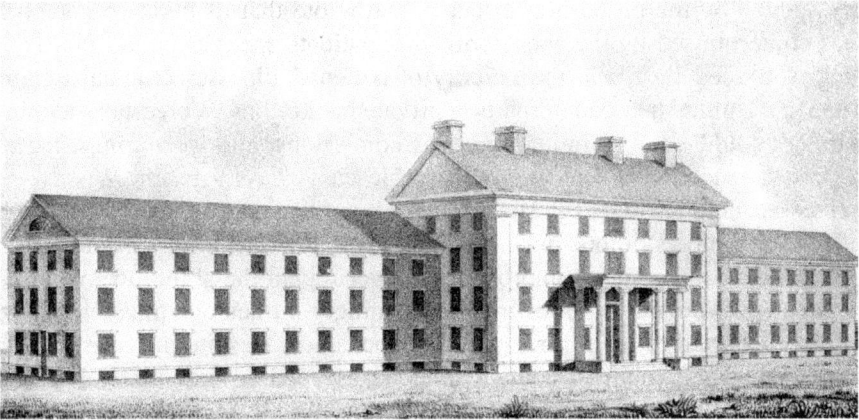

Figure 0.2 The Worcester State Hospital Pictured around the Time of Its Construction in 1833. Pendleton's Lithography, Boston. Courtesy of the Worcester Historical Museum.

The superintendent played an essential role in moral treatment, serving not only as the head of staff and primary medical officer but also as a moral guide to the asylum "family." Samuel B. Woodward, who served as the physician at the Hartford Retreat, a private Connecticut asylum that was modeled after the York Retreat, was an ideal choice (Cherry 1989: 170; Eaton 1957: 61–66). Although not a Quaker himself, Woodward ascribed to the model of treatment practiced at the Quaker-run institution, believing that "the benign influence of sympathy and compassion" exerted by the asylum was capable of "disarm[ing] [the] fury" of the "maniac" and transforming him into "a quiet, peaceable, intelligent and reasonable being" (Annual Report 1841: 70). Woodward also held progressive beliefs surrounding prison reform, public education, and intemperance, which he believed "should rather be considered as a disease than as a crime" (Woodward 1831). As one of his first actions as Worcester's superintendent, Woodward accepted the commitment of Howard Trask, a notorious lunatic who was "looked upon as a Demon" and had been "exhibited as a show" in the villages of Massachusetts (Woodward 1832). In March 1832, Woodward proudly reported to Horace Mann that Trask was "without chains[,] associating with our better class of patients[,] as yet perfectly quiet and peaceable" (ibid.). Woodward's success in pacifying Trask represented a bold illustration of the promises of moral treatment that reiterated the apocryphal scene in which Philippe Pinel—the father of moral treatment in France—liberated the inmates of the Salpêtrière Asylum from their chains (Browne 1837: 138).

Yet Woodward's descriptions of the asylum, widely disseminated through his annual reports, also testify to the difficulty of realizing the ideals of moral treatment on a consistent basis. Recognizing that the asylum would be "judged by the proportion of cures," he wrote that its curative potential was compromised by the short terms that patients spent at the hospital, the lack of trained staff, and the severity of patients' illnesses (Annual Report 1833: 3). Unlike their counterparts at private institutions, Worcester's administrators could not discriminate in their admissions, and were compelled to accept "a selection of the most deplorable cases." As a result, Woodward expressed the fear that "the Hospital will soon become the mere receptacle of foreign paupers, idiots, imbeciles, and incurables" (ibid.: 8). Some would not recover; others might improve, but never regain the ability to live independently. Even Trask, following his seemingly miraculous transformation, quickly reverted to his former pattern of behavior. Despite the construction of a specialized room to contain him, he escaped several times over the next decade ("Bill for Building Trask's Room" 1833; "Trask Caught" 1833; Annual Report 1844: 39).

Administrators learned just how drastically they had underestimated the magnitude of their responsibility when the hospital reached full capacity within its first few months of operation (Annual Report 1833). The resultant straining of its resources undermined the aims of moral treatment—namely, individualized care and healthy, comfortable living conditions—and was most frequently cited as the main factor threatening the success of its mission. Administrators framed the solution to this problem in architectural terms, believing that the spatial dimensions of the asylum were key to its efficacy. The first addition to the Worcester State Hospital, which appended two additional wings and nearly doubled its capacity, was completed in 1836 (Annual Report 1836). Over the next decades, administrators would continuously entreat the state legislature for funds to construct additional space for patients, as well as separate accommodations for imbeciles, the violently insane, African Americans, and immigrants, which they believed were necessary to uphold order and enable medical classification (Annual Report 1834, 1845; Trustees' Notes 1833). Despite these challenges, the Worcester State Hospital held a reputation as a "model institution" for its first few decades (Annual Report 1845: 5). Through the dissemination of its annual reports and visitations by physicians from other states, the design and administration of the hospital were highly influential, and the majority of American "mental hospitals built after 1833 were modeled after Worcester" (Grob 1966: 34). The optimistic attitude of its administrators reflected the dominance of a so-called "cult of curability" in the treatment of insanity, a natural outgrowth of the optimism of the age (Jarvis 1865: 255; Eaton 1957: 144; Grob 1966: 74). Woodward's statistics, published in each annual report, corroborated beliefs in curability, indicating a 90% cure rate for patients admitted within six months of the onset of symptoms (Annual Report 1834: 85).

Over the course of the nineteenth century, however, it became painfully obvious that the hospital was not nearly as effective as had been anticipated. Growth of the native population, a massive influx of immigrants, and the rising public image of the asylum as a therapeutic—or at least respectable— repository for insane family members combined to swell the number of new admissions (figure 0.3). Prior to 1870, the hospital rarely received more than 300 admissions annually; after 1890, this number never again dipped below 400, reaching a peak of 970 in 1919. At the same time, the asylum retained a steadily growing class of "incurables": chronically ill patients who remained at the asylum for years or decades. In 1877 Pliny Earle, superintendent of the Northampton State Hospital, dealt a damaging blow to the legitimacy of the Worcester State Hospital with his treatise *The Curability of Insanity*, in which he asserted that the published statistics of Worcester and other institutions had dramatically misrepresented the number of cures (Earle 1877, 1887). In fact, Earle wrote, the proportion of asylum patients who were "curable" was much smaller than originally projected and was growing smaller (Earle 1887: 42). Earle's rhetoric would become canonical of a new generation of psychiatrists whose belief in the promises of moral treatment had soured into "therapeutic pessimism" (Gamwell and Tomes 1984: 119; Morrissey and Goldman 1980: 62). Gerald Grob attributes the "retrogress[ion]" of the state hospital in the second half of the nineteenth century to a maelstrom of

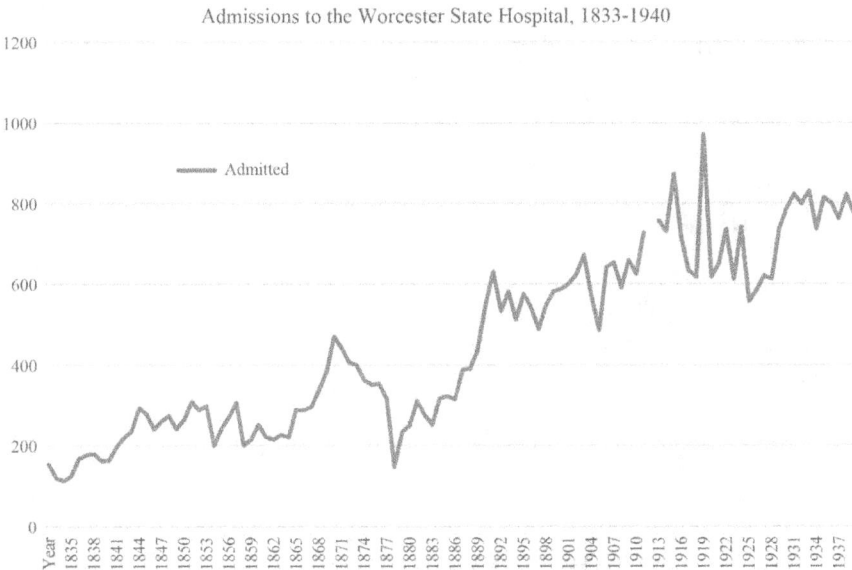

Figure 0.3 Admissions to the Worcester State Hospital, 1833-1940. The break in the line indicates a year for which data is not available. Created by the author.

factors—including a growing "sense of complacency, the belief that progress was determined by inexorable historical laws, social and class tensions, and religious and ethnic conflicts"—that culminated in an overall "decline in confidence of human ability to cope with mental disease" (Grob 1966: 115). While the early proponents of moral treatment had viewed lunatics as the victims of environmental factors, later psychiatrists were increasingly liable to attribute insanity to degeneration and heredity: a physical and moral corruption that was both intrinsic and irremediable.

The statistics collected by administrators seemed to corroborate Earle's claims (figure 0.4). Under Woodward's tenure in the 1830s and 1840s, the percentage of patients discharged "recovered" was consistently above 50% (with the exception of 1841, in which 49.16% were "recovered"). While this number sank slightly following Woodward's retirement, it remained between 30 and 75% throughout the mid-nineteenth century. Beginning in the 1870s, coincident with the rise of "therapeutic pessimism," the number of recoveries began to fall; at the same time, the percentage of patients who were discharged "not improved" increased. The inflation of the numbers of "not improved," particularly in certain years (such as 1853 and 1886) was partly a product of efforts to reduce the population by offloading "incurable" yet quiet patients to other institutions, such as poorhouses and prisons. The relinquishing of patients to nontherapeutic settings reflected administrators' beliefs that they were beyond hope of recovery.

The increase in the percentage of "incurable" cases coincided with a rising proportion of pauper patients at the hospital, a trend that served to further

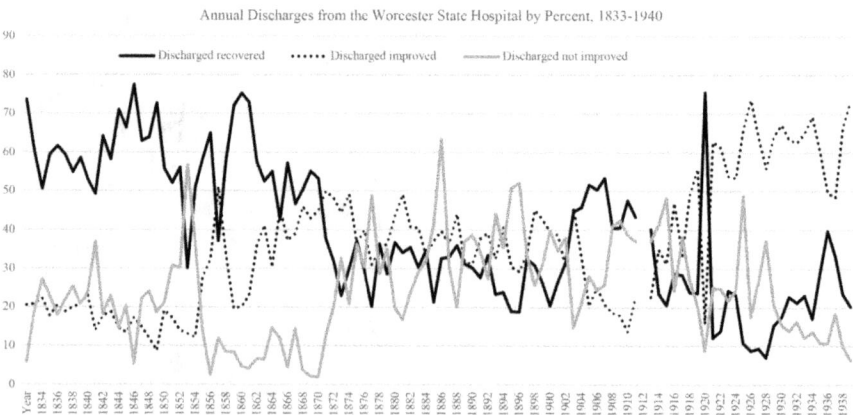

Figure 0.4 Annual Discharges from the Worcester State Hospital by Percent, Indicating a General Decline in the Percentage of Discharged Patients Who Were Considered "Recovered." The break in the line indicates a year for which data is not available. Created by the author.

entrench associations between poverty and insanity, as well as to undercut the public standing of the institution. In the first few decades of the hospital, the percentage of patients who were considered "paupers"—that is, residents of Massachusetts who were supported by their respective towns, or in the case of immigrants, by the state—comprised between 60 and 70% of the total population. The remainder were private patients whose treatment was underwritten by their families or friends. Beginning in the 1870s, this percentage began to increase, rising from around 60% in the early years of the decade to 80% by its end and reaching 85% in the 1880s, 90% by 1910, and 95% by 1920. The reputation of the hospital as a pauper institution likely served to dissuade families with the means to afford treatment from housing their insane relatives there, thus further deepening the divide between state hospitals and their private counterparts and depriving the former of a much-needed source of revenue. The state was similarly less inclined to invest its resources in an institution that had appeared to have become "the mere receptacle of foreign paupers, idiots, imbeciles, and incurables" that Woodward had foreseen.

Thus the deterioration of the "cult of curability" was instantiated in the decay of its central figure, the asylum itself. Year after year, state appropriations fell below the amount needed to expand the hospital in proportion to its growing population or to keep its existing buildings in repair. With a patient population more than double that of its capacity, under the care of only three medical officers, the hospital could hardly expect to maintain the quality of treatment it had offered in the 1830s. Administrators bemoaned the fact that "[o]ur Hospital at Worcester has not only ceased to be regarded as a model institution, but it has fallen into the rear rank in the march of improvement" (Annual Report 1853: 17). Their complaints were corroborated by the Massachusetts State Commission of Lunacy, whose 1855 investigation of the hospital discovered "unsatisfactory" drainage, obsolete ventilation and heating systems, and severe structural deficiencies (Jarvis 1855). Lead investigator Edward Jarvis suggested that the property be sold and the proceeds used to fund a "new and satisfactory hospital with all the recent improvements" (ibid.: 182). Instead, the state authorized the construction of a second state hospital at Northampton, completed in 1858. Despite providing accommodations for hundreds of patients, this measure provided only a temporary reprieve, as both hospitals were quickly filled beyond capacity. The Worcester State Hospital would continue to operate in a state of worsening crowding and dereliction for the next two decades.

THE SECOND HOSPITAL

The second Worcester State Hospital, opened in 1877, was located in the eastern side of the city, as far as possible from its industrial and business districts. Constructed on the so-called "linear" or "Kirkbride" plan—named for superintendent of the Pennsylvania Hospital for the Insane, Dr. Thomas Story Kirkbride—the building consisted of two symmetrical wings that receded from the central administration building in a distinctive zigzag pattern (figure 0.5) (Annual Report 1877: 7; Kirkbride 1854). The monumentality of the second hospital, effected through its massive size and baroque ornament, durable materials and stately landscape, lent the institution an air of authority that was necessary to buttress its lofty pledge to rehabilitate minds through the manipulation of the environment (Yanni 2007). The structure formalized many of the early century's beliefs about mental illness, when therapeutic optimism was at its height, and was conceived quite literally a medical instrument; not just a place of cure, but a curative place: the arrangement and the material of the building intended to exert a force that operated specifically through the medium of the senses. However, this force was interpolated by many variables, including the turning of the paradigmatic tide away from therapeutic optimism, the continued inadequacy of state

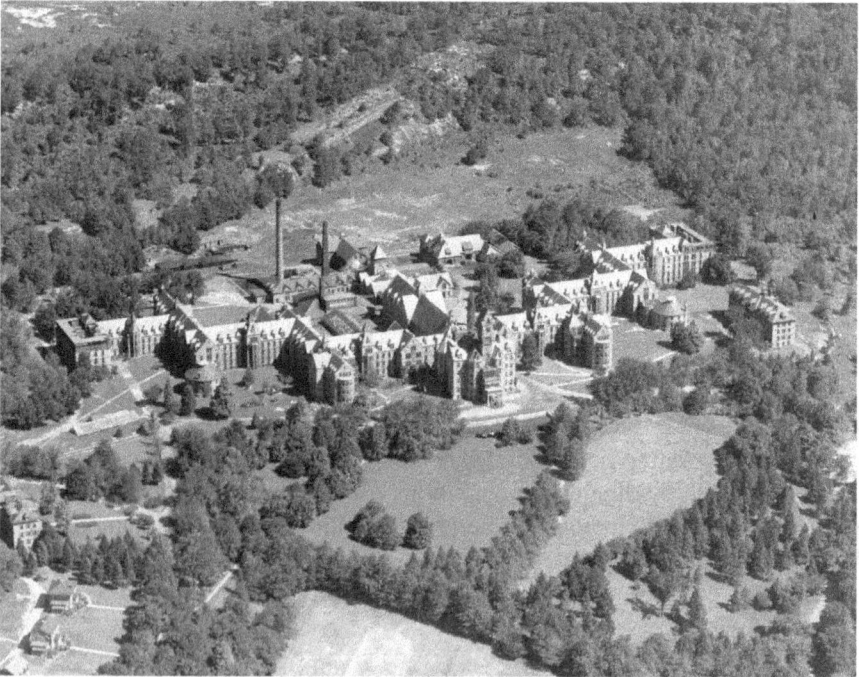

Figure 0.5 Aerial Photograph of the Second Worcester State Hospital Showing the Distinctive Receding Wings of the Kirkbride Plan. Paul Wentworth Savage, "Aerial photographs of Worcester and Worcester County, Massachusetts," 1927. Courtesy of the Worcester Historical Museum.

appropriations, and severe overcrowding, all of which inflected the sensory assemblage of the hospital.

While state-of-the-art at the time of its construction, the infrastructure of the second hospital quickly fell into obsolescence and disrepair. Administrators complained of the failing water supply and overburdened sewage system, inadequate facilities for bathing and dining, faulty electric wiring that posed the constant risk of fire, and a lack of sufficient refrigeration. An ever increasing amount of land was needed to meet the hospital's agricultural needs, yet the city continuously encroached on the hospital property, leading administrators to purchase a large farm in the neighboring town of Shrewsbury. Low wages and long work hours contributed to a high turnover among hospital staff and culminated in a 1902 nurses' strike. In addition to their own grievances, the strikers remonstrated on behalf of their patients, citing inedible food, lack of bedding, the proliferation of vermin, and neglect owing to insufficient staffing ("Nurses in rebellion" 1902; "Put out bag and baggage!" 1902; Annual Report 1902: 11–12). The patients in the crowded hospital, which lacked the space to impose a proper quarantine, were vulnerable to infectious disease, and their population was continuously ravaged by outbreaks of diphtheria, smallpox, influenza, scarlet fever, measles, and dysentery (Annual Report 1890).

Throughout the last decades of the nineteenth century, administrators complained that the "hospital is now so crowded with patients that officers are overwhelmed with routine duties," making it "impossible to give individual cases special care and attention" (Annual Report 1896: 5). Under such conditions, the character of the asylum inevitably shifted from the curative to the custodial, turning a once therapeutic institution into a "dumping ground for a heterogeneous mass of physical and mental wrecks" (Scull 1979: 194, 252). The recruitment of Dr. Ado Meyer as the hospital's first pathologist in 1895 was intended to reinvigorate the mission of the hospital through a new empirical approach to insanity. Under Meyer's brief but impactful leadership, the hospital established research laboratories to study mental disease and its treatment (Annual Report 1895: 15; Annual Report 1902: 7). Administrators reported that as a result of this "new departure," a "scientific spirit and *atmosphere* pervade[d]" the hospital (Annual Report 1899: 7). While research at Worcester would continue into the twentieth century and ultimately make significant contributions to the science of mental health, the new ethos of the hospital served to dehumanize patients, who were treated largely as guinea pigs, subjected to experimental testing and treatment against their will.

After Meyer's departure in 1902, Worcester "sunk [back] into warehousing mediocrity" (Callaway 2007: 132). By 1908, the building was packed with over 1,200 patients: more than double the number it was originally designed to accommodate (Annual Report 1908: 7). Under these conditions, administrators adopted a disorganized and ad hoc approach to the treatment of insanity that would later be termed "therapeutic eclecticism" (Martin 2007). Unlike moral treatment, this approach had no central philosophy or theoretical structure, but rather encompassed a variety of therapies that were applied with little understanding of whether or how they might work, including hydrotherapy, shock therapy, hormone therapy, psychoanalysis, and lobotomy (El-Hai 2005: 211; Callaway 2007).

As early as 1914, administrators questioned the scale of the hospital's inpatient population, stating that "many persons now in institutions, while obviously insane, may profitably be returned to the community" (Annual Report 1914: 11). Over the next decades, they hired social workers and organized public programs and outpatient treatment centers to foster connections between the institution and the community, facilitate the reintegration of patients into society, and prevent the necessity of hospital treatment through early intervention and education. Despite these efforts, the patient population continued to grow, even as its public image began to decline. By the mid-twentieth century, the Worcester State Hospital and many similar institutions were experiencing a crisis of identity in a world that increasingly viewed them as retrograde and barbaric "human warehouses" (Morrissey, Goldman, and Klerman 1980: 1). Investigative works on asylums—including the 1967 film *Titicut Follies*, which exposed the neglect and abuse of patients at the Bridgewater State Hospital in Bridgewater, Massachusetts—scandalized the public and led to calls for reform.

Deinstitutionalization was viewed as a "remedy for 'institutionalism,' the social-psychiatric syndrome associated with prolonged exposure to a debilitating custodial environment" (Morrissey et al. 1980: 9). The emergence of the first antipsychotic drugs, which controlled the symptoms of severe mental illness, further undermined the perceived necessity of inpatient treatment. Accordingly, the 1960s and 1970s witnessed the release of hundreds of thousands of patients and the shuttering of state hospitals across the country. The first state to institute a systematic program of institutional treatment for the insane, Massachusetts was also one of the last to deinstitutionalize, a program largely driven by the unilateral actions made by its Republican governor over the objections of the Democratic legislature and hospital employees (Upshur et al. 1997: 206). Between 1991 and 1993, ten institutions were shuttered. While the Worcester State Hospital continued to operate, absorbing a portion of the patients who remained in state custody after the closure of other institutions, it did so on an increasingly smaller scale. Today, the Worcester State Hospital—now known as the Worcester Recovery Center and Hospital—holds the capacity for 320 patients, a small fraction of the 3,000 it accommodated in 1950 (Myerson 1980: 114).

Even before the negative consequences of deinstitutionalization became evident, patient advocates and mental health professionals questioned the decision to systematically dismantle the country's state hospital system. While acknowledging the faults of the system, they have pointed to the failure of state and federal governments to provide for the hundreds of thousands of former patients who have been shuffled from "back wards" to "back alleys" (Goldman 1980: 134). Some of these individuals had lived in institutions for years or even decades and lacked the skills and resources to function in society. Once released, many became homeless or were incarcerated. Today, the majority of inpatient mental health care in the United States takes place in prisons, rather than in hospitals (Kim 2016). Critics of deinstitutionalization argue that the repudiation of the asylum model has resulted in a "collective amnesia" whereby the hard-won lessons of years of institutional practice have been lost (Etzioni 1975: 12). In the words of Oliver Sacks, "We forgot the benign aspects of asylums, or perhaps we felt we could no longer pay for them" (Sacks 2009: 5).

This book represents part of a recent effort to re-examine the asylum in light of its original promise and early successes. My purpose is not to summarily reject the work of social control theorists or to undermine the many painful testimonies to the negative effects of institutionalization. Rather, my purpose is to consider *both* the "benign aspects" and the failures of the asylum simultaneously, to allow these contradictions to coexist, and to mobilize their disharmony to yield a more nuanced and complete understanding of the asylum and its legacy. Dr. Enoch Callaway, who served as a medical resident at Worcester State Hospital in the 1940s, believed that the asylum was "both a snake pit and a model hospital, a safe house and a warehouse" (Callaway 2007: 6). My analysis is situated in this chasm between the asylum's original mission and its subsequent failures. I argue that the framework of the senses provides a means of transcending previous models of asylum historiography that have focused on a linear narrative of the asylum's emergence, development, and collapse, as well as works of scholarship that seek to either condemn or vindicate the asylum. Instead, a sensory framework offers the opportunity to redirect attention toward the human element of asylums by articulating the lived experiences that emerged in the interface between the mind, the body, and the institution.

ANTHROPOLOGY AND ARCHAEOLOGY OF THE SENSES

The historical archaeology of institutions is an emergent subfield that offers a set of tools for examining the power dynamics of total institutions through the materiality of lived experience. Historical archaeologists have taken a variety of different approaches, ranging from excavation and architectural survey to the systematic study of architectural plans, case notes, and other documentary evidence. What binds them together beneath the auspices of a single discipline is what Michael Shanks describes as an "archaeological sensibility": not a single method or theory, but "a pervasive set of *attitudes* towards traces and remains, towards memory, time and temporality, the fabric of history" (Shanks 2012: 25, emphasis added). As Benjamin Alberti writes, the exercise of an archaeological sensibility involves the application of "skill and discernment" to evidence from the past: the "care and attentiveness that archaeologists bring to their practical work in order to bring out meaning" (Alberti 2018).

Accordingly, the objective of the historical archaeology of institutions is not only to produce new bodies of evidence but also to develop new ways of conceptualizing institutions. Running through these studies are the themes of *dissonance*—between what the institution was supposed to have been and what it turned out to be, and between traditional narratives and the evidence that archaeology can provide—and *ambiguity*: the blurry spaces where the narratives produced by various lines of evidence diverge (Leone and Crosby 1987; Andrén 1998). Historical archaeologists studying institutions seek to counterbalance the distortions of the historical record by reanimating the other half of the "dynamic interplay of authority and resistance" that structured the institution (Surface-Evans 2016: 586); yet they also acknowledge that the relationships represented in the institution are more complex than this simple binary, looking to the "physical experience of confinement as a way to emphasize the *diversity* of experiences" (Casella 2009: 26).

Archaeological studies of asylums have targeted specific points of dissonance and ambiguity in the evidence surrounding these institutions. In her study of insane asylums in Australia, Tasmania, and Britain, Susan Piddock discovered a "sharp contrast between the world of ideas . . . and reality as built" (Piddock 2007: 18). While intended to provide a "comfortable and curative environment" that would offer a comprehensive set of therapeutic resources, in practice, such institutions were poorly organized, "cold and unwelcoming," and offered few means of therapy or even provisions for ordinary amusement (Piddock 2003: 47, 2007: 220). Similarly, in her archaeological investigation of the Royal Edinburgh Asylum, Joanna Dawson found "huge differences in the treatment of private and pauper patients"—specifically in the style and type of ceramics and correspondent dietary options—that controvert the democratizing rhetoric upon which the institution was founded (Dawson 2003).

The work of Dawson and Piddock on insane asylums has no equivalent in the United States. While historical archaeologists have studied a variety of American total institutions—including poor farms, almshouses, houses of reform, internment camps, and boarding schools—little attention has been dedicated to asylums for the insane (Spencer-Wood and Baugher 2001). Notably, the most extensive study of American insane asylums as artifacts comes not from the discipline of historical archaeology but from architectural history. In *The Architecture of Madness* (2007), Carla Yanni takes the structures and spaces of American asylums as the object of her analysis. Like Piddock, she explores the disjuncture between the idealized template for the asylum and the "messy" realities into which it was translated (Yanni 2007: 14). In doing so, Yanni demonstrates the value of a material and spatial approach to understanding both the promise and the failure of a curative program that was predicated on the manipulation of bodies and minds through the built environment.

As a discipline that has traditionally positioned itself as the study "of small things forgotten," of everyday experience, and of ordinary and/or marginalized people (Deetz 1996), historical archaeology holds the potential to reanimate the complexities of the asylum dynamic. While this lens has been successfully applied to studies of the asylum in other countries, additional study is needed to elucidate the power structures and historical contingencies of American asylums, which followed a unique ideological and architectural trajectory. This book applies the interdisciplinary methodology of historical archaeology—with its focus on context, power, and experience; appreciation for the nuances and ambiguity of sources; and use of material and spatial evidence—to address three major questions, representing three distinct subfields of anthropology.

Medical anthropology provides a means for framing the complexities of the illness experience as they were situated within the asylum and its sociocultural landscape, posing the question: How is illness understood and experienced in context? Medical anthropologists problematize the conception of illness as fundamentally biological, presenting an alternative paradigm—predicated on the contingencies of cultural context and individual experience—which "challenges biomedical hegemony" (Scheper-Hughes 1989: 67). Concepts such as Kleinman's "social suffering" and Biehl's "social psychosis" recast illness as biocultural rather than strictly biological or social in nature (Kleinman et al. 1997; Biehl 2013). Medical anthropologists have argued that while "madness is real," it is also deeply "involved with our social fabric" (Luhrmann 2001: 17); accordingly, it must be contextualized within its historical and spatial setting. This book contributes to the medical anthropological scholarship on illness in two ways. First, by historicizing the presiding biomedical model of mental illness that structures present-day psychiatry, a field which derived from asylum medicine. And second, by lending a material and spatial dimension to the contextualization of mental illness, which medical anthropologists argue is experienced through bodily engagement with and in the surrounding social and physical environment.

These bodily experiences may be accessed through an engagement with phenomenology, a field which asks: How is the environment perceived and experienced? Phenomenology works from the premise that "the built world presents a philosophical problem, or better, that it demands philosophical reflection" (Dodd 2017). Scholars of anthropology, history, and architectural history acknowledge that "the treatment of the insane is conducted not only *in,* but *by* the asylum" (Yanni 2007). Given the intention with which asylum architects worked to invest their curative environments with agentive power, it is striking that studies of the asylum have tended to neglect the materiality of the asylum itself (Piddock 2007; Yanni 2007). This neglect is indicative of a larger tendency within the social sciences, including archaeology, to treat the physical world as an *expression* of culture, which is "somehow 'prior' or detached from matter" (Olsen 2010). In contrast, phenomenology conceptualizes artifacts, landscapes, and the built environment as "social facts" in themselves (Durkheim 1951; Ashmore and Knapp 1999; Tilley 1994; Gosden 1994). While both asylum medicine and phenomenology foreground the agency of the environment in their constructions of reality, nineteenth-century alienists reified this dualism, suggesting that environment was a separate entity that controlled the psyches and behavior of the people lodged within it. In contrast, phenomenology—like medical anthropology—problematizes the Cartesian dualism between mind and matter (Husserl 1960; Marsh 1988; Olsen 2010). Phenomenologists suggest that the environment possesses agentive properties precisely because environment and people, and matter and intellect, are *not* separate entities, but rather represent "entangled beings" and "engaged subjects" that collaborate in the production of action and meaning (Olsen 2010). By mobilizing the senses as a framework for articulating the interface between the asylum and the social actors who populated it, this book offers a new way of conceptualizing this entanglement.

Archaeologists have used phenomenology to understand how power is enacted, disseminated, and resisted through the entanglement of the body and environment in the realm of everyday action (Heidegger 1971; Gosden 1994; Johnson 2012; Joyce 2005). This work connects phenomenological archaeology to the anthropological interest in discipline, surveillance, and power, which centers the question: How is power enacted, maintained, and resisted? Anthropologists still draw upon Foucauldian theories of social control in describing how the historical asylum functioned as a "site of moral synthesis" and how psychiatry perpetuates the asylum's role as an "agent of reality" (Foucault 1971, 2005; De Cunzo 1995; Das 2016; Beisaw and Gibb 2009). However, these theories have been modulated and expanded by critiques across the social sciences, including archaeology (Luhrmann 2001;

Mills 2000; Murat 2014; Porter 2002; Reiss 2008; Spencer-Wood 2010; Piddock 2007; Hamlett 2013). Such critiques lend a much-needed degree of complexity to the grand, schematizing narratives that characterized the first generation of asylum historiography. They have balanced the traditionally "top-down" perspective on asylums with a "bottom-up" approach taken from the "patient's view," illuminating individual agency and acts of resistance (Porter 1985; Smith 2008; Morrison 2016; Bivins and Pickstone 2007; Scott 1990; Reaume 2000). They have also identified the historical contingencies that shaped experiences in various asylums across space and time, demonstrating the difficulty of generalizing about "the asylum" as a singular entity (Alleridge 1985; Digby 1985; Andrews 1998; Davis 2008; De Cunzo 2009; Baugher 2009). In contextualizing the experience of mental illness as a function of the particular sensory dimensions of its built environment, I build upon anthropological approaches that foreground materiality, spatiality, local contingencies, and lived experience as central forces in the dynamic interplay of power within the total institution.

Finally, the senses offer a novel instrument for furthering the project of historical archaeology to conceptualize the everyday entanglement of the body and environment in the historical institution (Gosden 1994; Johnson 2012). Rather than invoking traditional concepts of "systems, networks, or social structures," I draw from recent work in archaeology and ethnography that seeks to "address the sensory deficiencies in archaeology" (Sorensen 2015; Day 2013). By conceptualizing the asylum as a "sensorial assemblage," comprised of a heterogeneity of bodily experiences refracted through the perspectives of various social actors, this book departs from traditional narratives that collapse the intricacies of the asylum into generalized schemas of domination and resistance (Hamilakis 2014). At the same time, it liberates the asylum from linear narratives of emergence, development, and decline, arguing that the "sensorial flows" of the asylum are inherently "multitemporal in nature," as trends in its therapeutic program moved forward, backward, and cyclically in response to internal and external variables (ibid.). In doing so, it poses an intervention that departs from previous expositions of the asylum, which have tended to focus on either on a top-down model of power in the institution, or a bottom-up perspective that foregrounds patient agency. By using the senses as a framing device, I interweave the perspectives of the multiple actors implicated in the asylum, targeting the facet of lived experience that both connected and distinguished them: their senses.

Although all humans share the same sensory apparatus, the stimuli received through the senses is mediated by social, cultural, and individual variables. Recent works of history and archaeology have begun to explore "the role of the senses in *framing* perceptual experience in accordance with socially prescribed norms" (Classen 1997: 401), arguing that the senses are not simply a passive mechanism for perceiving the world but may be actively mobilized as instruments of power and control. Governed by state and medical authorities who believed they were charged with the authority to define and enforce the laws of nature, the asylum was a "sensorial-affective regime" designed to reform the insane subject through the manipulation of the sensory environment (Hamilakis 2014: 2). It is possible to analyze the sensorial assemblage of the asylum solely through the lens of social control; yet to do so would underestimate the significance of alternative sensory frameworks and their dynamic interaction with the dominant discourse. Following Hamilakis, I target the "tension between the anarchic and messy world of the senses, and the often politically motivated attempts by various people and groups to regulate and channel sensorial experience, often using material culture and physical and built space" (ibid.). These points of slippage abound in the history of the asylum, as authorities attempted to force their patients' sensory experiences into alignment with the institution's sensorial regime only to collide against the persistent efforts of patients in creating and maintaining their own "worlds of sense" (Classen 1997).

METHODOLOGY

Archaeologists who study historical lunatic asylums face many practical challenges. The state hospitals of Massachusetts exist today in a range of different conditions, reflecting the vagaries of their use, ownership, and preservation. Some, like the Medfield State Hospital, have been kept relatively intact, although vacant and vulnerable to decay. Others, like the Tewksbury State Hospital, have been updated to meet the standards of a modern facility and continue to operate as inpatient treatment centers (albeit on a much smaller scale than they once did). A larger number of nineteenth-century state hospitals have been sold to developers and partially or completely demolished to make way for new construction. The present condition of the Worcester State Hospital represents a patchwork of these different outcomes. The majority of the once 500-acre property—including its former agricultural fields and sweeping front lawn and gardens—has been subdivided and sold. The gradual abandonment of the second hospital building—that is, the Kirkbride complex, built in 1877—began in 1957, when 860 of the hospital's 2,600 patients were moved to the newly constructed Bryan Building, adjacent to the nineteenth-century structure (Morrissey and Goldman 1980: 86). By the 1980s, the entire patient population—which then numbered less than 500—had been transferred to the Bryan Building (ibid.). The Kirkbride was vacant yet largely intact when it was devastated by fire in 1991. In 2008, most of what remained of the nineteenth-century building was demolished to make way for a new (and significantly smaller) hospital. The destruction of the Kirkbride, a structure listed on the National Register of Historic Places since 1993, was widely protested (Southwick 2012). The campaign of local activists was critical in saving two sections from demolition: the iconic central clock tower and the Hooper Turret, a round, open-plan structure originally designed for the accommodation of suicidal female patients (Kane 2015).

As I discuss in chapter 1, the Hooper Turret—along with its counterpart on the male side of the complex, the Gage Turret—represented a novel approach to the treatment of insanity through a specially designed architecture of surveillance. My original plans for this project included an investigation of the role of visibility—both the visibility of the environment to patients and the visibility of patients to caretakers and to each other—in shaping experiences of confinement in the Hooper Turret, using viewshed analysis and architectural survey. However, as the best-laid plans have a tendency to do, this fell through. While initially receptive to my proposal to survey the building, the Massachusetts State Department of Mental Health rescinded its permission to access the Hooper Turret, citing safety concerns. These concerns were not unreasonable, as the building has been vacant, without regular maintenance, for over 30 years. The amount of damage inflicted by the 1991 fire on the Hooper Turret is unclear (some areas of the Kirkbride were relatively untouched, while others were completely gutted). Although the building has not been open to visitors in decades, I was familiar with several photographers who accessed the building illicitly before the remainder of the Kirkbride was demolished in 2008 (their photographs are widely available online). I contacted one of these photographers, who told me that some of the floors in the Worcester State Hospital had completely collapsed or were in imminent danger of doing so when he visited in the mid-2000s. Legal issues surrounding the impending sale of a section of the remaining hospital property to developers in 2017, as well as concerns for patient privacy, further restricted my access. I was able to visit the site through contacts with members of the hospital staff, but these visits were largely confined to the interiors of the current hospital and the area immediately surrounding it.

With these limitations in mind, it was necessary to approach this project with a spirit of creativity, resourcefulness, and a keen awareness of the defining attributes of historical archaeology. As Susan Piddock writes, "excavation is not an essential part of archaeological practice"; rather, it is "the questions being asked"—the "attitudes" of "archaeological sensibility"—that distinguish historical archaeology as a discipline (Piddock 2009: 22). Historical archaeologists treat buildings and landscapes as artifacts, which function both as a material record of their use over time and as agents that actively intervene in the unfolding of events. My methodology proceeded from this conception of the asylum as both accretional and agentive in nature. Although devised for a distinct purpose—to cure insanity—once that design was given material dimensions, the Worcester State Hospital took on an agency of its own, which exerted a material and ideational force on its inhabitants, and in turn was shaped by these inhabitants' agentive acts. In my investigation, I targeted this "dialectical relationship in institutional change," which operates foremost in the realm of everyday experience (Beisaw and Gibb 2009: 4). In doing so, I sought to practice what Lu Ann De Cunzo describes as a "holistic" and "intertextual" approach, which "explores what people did in each space, when and how, with what, with whom," and most importantly, *"why":* an "experiential and processual archaeology of the mind, spirit, and body" (De Cunzo 2009: 209–210).

To articulate and organize this practice, I posed the following questions:

1. How was the building and its landscape of the Worcester State Hospital *designed* to exert a therapeutic influence on patients through the realm of sensory experience?
2. How did the construction and administration of the asylum *in reality* shape the sensory experiences of its patients?

To answer question 1, I needed to understand the decisions made in the construction of the Worcester State Hospital as well as the local, sociocultural, and intellectual contexts that framed those decisions. In addition to a broad range of nineteenth-century sources relating to health and medicine, physiology and the senses, insanity and deviance, and domestic and public architecture, I drew upon the genre of asylum literature that emerged in the early nineteenth century to furnish physicians, administrators, and architects with guidelines and specifications for the "ideal" institution. This literature includes Samuel Tuke's *Practical Hints on the Construction and Economy of Pauper Lunatic Asylums* (1815), W. A. F. Browne's *What Asylums Were, Are, and Ought to Be* (1837), John Conolly's *Construction and Government of Lunatic Asylums and Hospitals for the Insane* (1847), and Thomas Kirkbride's *On the Construction, Organization, and General Arrangements for Hospitals for the Insane* (1854). These works enabled me to situate the Worcester State Hospital within the wider movement of nineteenth-century institutions for the insane, as well as to understand the influence that Worcester—as one of the earliest state hospitals in the United States—exerted on the course of asylum history.

To understand the design of the two nineteenth-century iterations of the Worcester State Hospital, I consulted documents at the Massachusetts State Archives, including a collection of contracts, receipts, and specifications relating to the construction of the first hospital on Summer Street, which itemized materials with rigorous precision, down to the number of bricks and nails that were ordered; the original foundation plans for the second Worcester State Hospital, held at the Worcester Historical Museum; and a large variety of written descriptions, photographs, and maps held at repositories across the state. In keeping with my theoretical framework, I looked for evidence that would help me to conceptualize the functioning of the asylum as a sensory environment, asking: What kind of sensory encounters was it intended to enable? What kinds of sensory encounters was it intended to inhibit? And how did these intentions articulate within the paradigm of moral treatment and within broader medical and cultural understandings of the relationship between environment and human beings, mind and body?

To answer question 2, I looked for evidence of the ways in which the hospital was operated and altered over time, and of the effects these practices had on patients' sensory experiences. Many scholars have described the difficulty of accessing the experiences of patients in historical institutions and the limitations of the existing evidence (Porter 1985; Andrews 1998; Morrison 2016; Smith 2008). "To discern the small voice" of the institutionalized patient of the nineteenth century "means coming to terms with the history that silenced it" (Swartz 2005: 517). The authors of first-person asylum narratives represent a select group of individuals who tended to be more privileged, educated, and mentally stable than the average patient, and thus were able to make their voices heard. Nonetheless, historians have managed to salvage valuable insights from patient accounts, as well as from letters, case notes, and other materials documenting patients' attitudes and behavior, in order to extend and challenge traditional conceptions of confinement in nineteenth-century institutions, including the Gloucester Asylum in England (Smith 2008), the Gartnavel Royal Asylum (Andrews 1998; Morrison 2016), and the Royal Edinburgh Asylum (Beveridge 1997). In my investigation, these first-person accounts, which were written from the point of view of individuals who were immersed in the sensory domain of the nineteenth-century asylum, serve as a foundational point of entry into the lived experience of confinement.

I was able to identify four patient accounts from the Worcester State Hospital in the nineteenth century: two accounts published anonymously in Worcester newspapers in 1844; Charles Foster's *Poetry Written By A Man After Being Kept Nearly Eight Years in the Worcester Insane Asylum* (1874); and *False Imprisonment of Elizabeth R. Hill* (1881). In addition to these Worcester-specific texts, I consulted the accounts of patients confined to contemporary state hospitals, including Nellie Bly (Blackwell's Island), Ebenezer Haskell (Pennsylvania Hospital), Isaac Hunt (Maine State Hospital), Elizabeth Packard (Jacksonville Insane Asylum), Moses Swan (Troy Lunatic Asylum and Brattleborough Asylum), Charles Henry Turner (Taunton Lunatic Hospital), Clifford Beers (Connecticut State Hospital and

the Hartford Retreat), and three patients from the McLean Asylum: Lydia
Denny, Robert Fuller, and Elizabeth Stone.

While these accounts were essential in delineating certain aspects of
patients' experience, they do not on their own provide a "holistic" view of
the dimensions of sensory confinement in the Worcester State Hospital, nor
enable the type of "intertextual" analysis—which is predicated on the juxtaposition of multiple viewpoints and types of evidence—that is fundamental
to the practice of historical archaeology. Accordingly, to supplement and
inform my reading of patients' writings, I looked for additional points of
access into the sensory dimensions of everyday life, where I might discover
small pieces of information—such as the design of the hospital's windows,
the arrangements made for sewage and ventilation, the use of bells and
buzzers, and the materials used in the walls and floors—that individually
constitute only trivia, but could be combined to render a multidimensional
conception of the asylum as sensorial assemblage. I studied the annual
reports of the Worcester State Hospital, which describe both the larger
executive decisions involved in the government of the asylum and the minutiae of everyday life, such as patients' diet, their recreational activities, the
books they read, and the number of socks they knitted. I read the accounts
of trustees who were tasked with visiting the hospital each month in order
to assess patients' living conditions; perused the pages of a friendship album
written and illustrated by a young woman working as a chamber maid in the
1840s; and immersed myself in the voluminous archives of Dr. Samuel B.
Woodward at the American Antiquarian Society. I consulted the hospital's
System of Regulations and *Hymns for the Hospital Chapel;* hunted down
descriptions of the building and landscape by nineteenth-century visitors and
features in the local newspapers; and sought out every graphic representation of the hospital I could find, ranging from photographs and illustrations
to postcards and commemorative plates. In comparing these multiple bodies
of evidence, I looked for sites of both agreement and discord; places where
the voices of one source either agreed or diverged with another; as well as
points of agreement and disjuncture between the "rhetoric" and the "reality"
of asylum life.

The framework of sensory experience and the methodology of historical
archaeology furnish the means for a synthesis that surpasses the limitations of
any one source or method. This process of searching, discovery, and assembly requires a degree of creativity, as well as an understanding of the inherent limitations of the archaeological imagination, yet when performed with a
critical and exhaustive approach, it can yield novel insights into overlooked
dimensions of the past. These "simple details of past experience" (Deetz
1996) lend a much-needed degree of texture to understandings of historical
institutions and hold the potential to significantly expand and even contest

existing narratives, with crucial implications for our understanding of modern society.

CHAPTER OVERVIEW

Most scholarly studies of the asylum follow a linear model, tracing the history of the institution from its promising early beginnings to its ultimate failure. While useful for understanding the transformation of the asylum over time, linear histories have had the unintended consequence of formulating an asylum narrative that is both monolithic—suggesting that asylums as a whole followed a broad downward arc from their idealistic conception to their repudiation— and teleological, as the trajectory of the asylum seems to pitch inevitably toward the state in which state hospitals exist today: as "curious relics" of a less enlightened age (Annual Report 1858: 7). A study of the senses enables the reorganization of the events and experiences of asylum life according to a different framework, allowing for the juxtaposition across and within temporal contexts and prioritizing the textures and rhythms of everyday experiences.

In chapter one, I trace the material dimensions of the asylum and how they changed over time. The deterioration of the institution, while partly attributable to the strains of overcrowding and lack of financial resources, was as much a function of its creators' inflexibility and nearsightedness. The monumental and immobile design of both hospitals imposed limits on their uses that intruded into subsequent eras and created discord with new paradigms of treatment. Administrators struggled to adjust the rigid material-ity of the asylum to accommodate developments in psychiatry. On the other hand, patients proved remarkably resourceful in mobilizing this materiality to their own uses, imposing their own meanings and uses onto the asylum and asserting their power as agents in the creation and modification of its sensory assemblage.

In chapter two, I describe administrators' efforts to mobilize the optics of the asylum as a means of therapy. While the asylum as it was originally designed offered views of bucolic surroundings, access to natural light, and cheerful interiors, these resources were differentially distributed across time and space and between patient populations. Yet even those patients who *did* receive the best visual experiences that the hospital had to offer did not benefit in the ways administrators expected. As explained in their accounts, patients' perceptions of their surroundings derived not from an "objective" assessment of its visual stimuli but rather from the subjectivities through which those stimuli were refracted. Accordingly, the visual therapeutics of the asylum were experienced as an attempt at optical trickery that collapsed under the scrutiny of patients' perceptions.

In my chapter three, I describe the competing tactics exercised by administrators and patients in their struggle for the control over the asylum soundscape. While both iterations of the Worcester State Hospital were positioned
to escape the contaminating noises of the city, the asylum ultimately became
a city unto itself, crowding together large groups of people and generating the
conditions for the concentration and amplification of sound. Administrators'
tactics to induce quiet consisted of a combination of psychological intimidation and physical coercion. Conflating "quiet" with sanity, they failed to recognize the role their actions played in crushing patients' spirits and thereby
thwarting the asylum's therapeutic potential. To patients, the ability to make
themselves heard was crucial to maintaining their autonomy and served as
one of the few available vehicles for protest.

In chapter four, I recount administrators' campaigns to master the olfactory
domain of the asylum. Administrators conceptualized hygiene primarily as
a function of individual behavior, rather than as a social construct that was
intimately connected to structural inequalities and bourgeois conceptions of
moral purity. When the anticipated cures failed to materialize, administrators
responded by doubling down on their beliefs in individual defectiveness, to
which they added emergent concepts of degeneration and hereditary taint.
This pessimistic turn justified administrative actions that privileged the maintenance of order and authority over therapeutic interventions and empathetic
treatment. While the living conditions of the asylum were never optimal, they
sank to an atrocious state after administrators abandoned the premise that
their patients were capable of recovery and worthy of kindness.

Finally, in chapter five, I discuss the multiple meanings and uses of food
in the asylum and how they were intended to support—yet ultimately undermined—its therapeutic mission. Through the "conflation of natural laws" of
health with social norms, administrators transformed the realm of food into
a social theater for the performance of class- and gender-based roles (Tomes
1984: 87). The terroristic regime of forced feeding perverted the realm of
food into an arena of domination and resistance, while the hierarchical organization of labor served to define and entrench divisions between patients.
The mobilization of working-class, "incurable" patients as a semi-permanent
class of laborers directly opposed the therapeutic imperative of healing
patients in order to return them to the outside world. The clash between these
objectives meant that the asylum's curative mission was placed in competition with—and often in subordination to—the demands of production.

Because the separation of the senses by chapter tends to impede the discussion of the relationship *between* disparate sensory domains, in my conclusion
I address the concept of "intersensoriality": the ways in which the inputs
from different senses interact to create particular embodied experiences. I
describe the ways that patients marshaled their multiple senses to deconstruct

the rhetorical and disciplinary forces of the asylum and thereby critique its efficacy as a therapeutic instrument. Foremost among patients' critiques was the assertion that the asylum environment not only failed to improve their health, but was fundamentally *iatrogenic*, or productive of disease. In posing this argument, patients did not controvert the *premise* of the asylum, but rather its faulty execution. To judge by their accounts, and by the scholarship of historians who have grappled with the asylum in the wake of deinstitutionalization, the doctrine of moral treatment was never given the resources necessary for its proper implementation, outside of a few small-scale contexts in the early nineteenth century: including, Gerald Grob has argued, the Worcester State Hospital in its first decades, under Woodward's stewardship (Grob 1966). This dissonance between the potential of the asylum and the realities of institutional practice forms the basis for the "ambiguous legacy" of the asylum today (Morrissey and Goldman 1980).

NOTES

1. Haskell was eventually declared sane by the Court of Common Pleas and released.

2. This practice partly endured through the requirement that local towns and villages pay the bill for board and treatment of their respective pauper lunatics in the state asylum.

3. Although the York Retreat was not a pauper lunatic asylum, it employed the same window design that Tuke endorsed in *Practical Hints*.

Chapter 1

"Curious Relics" and "Drafty Corridors"

The Material World of the Asylum

The asylum was, first and foremost, a material object. No other feature played as significant a role in defining and materializing the theoretical aims and shaping the sensory experiences of its inhabitants as the building and its setting. Psychiatrists placed priority on the structure, layout, and material qualities of the asylum as embodiments of its therapeutic program (Callaway 2007: 168). While this emphasis on asylum design would come to be derided as "The Edifice Complex" by critics who accused administrators of squandering the potential of asylums as research laboratories, the idea that the built environment was a defining feature of experience and could be manipulated to produce certain effects—even radically transformative ones—was not unique to psychiatry. From ancient megalithic monuments to modern city planning, human beings have mobilized the agentive and semiotic powers of the built environment as a means of conveying meaning, embodying knowledge, and naturalizing ideologies.

The asylum as envisioned by psychiatrists was much more than a setting for the practice of moral treatment; it was primarily an *instrument* of that treatment. Together, the buildings and landscape of the asylum organized the spatial and temporal dimensions of everyday life, enabling the "choreographing of experiences" and the curation of sensory stimuli (Casella 2001: 50). The aim of this sensory management was not simply to provide an atmosphere that was conducive to recovery, but to exert a certain form of control over patients. Through "a moral architecture of enclosure, confinement, separation, isolation, articulation, and observation," the asylum engineered and enforced its own brand of discipline (De Cunzo 1995: 44), which targeted the interface between the material environment and the bodies that inhabited it. The asylum was invested with such power as a therapeutic agent that many psychiatrists believed that *the building alone* was capable of curing certain patients, without any additional interventions. As German physician and phrenologist J. G. Spurzheim observed, "patients violent in their families [often] become quiet as soon as they are confined in an asylum" (Spurzheim 1833: 200).

Psychiatric theory surrounding asylums resonated with popular ideologies surrounding residential architecture. "It is a solemn thing to build a house," architect E. C. Gardner wrote in *Homes and How to Make Them*. "You not only influence your fellow-men, but reveal your own character; for houses have a facial expression as marked as that of human beings" (Gardner 1874: 16–17). To psychiatrists, the asylum represented the "face" of their profession—a monument to the humanitarianism and progressivism of its founders—while its internal arrangements served as a metaphor for its theoretical organization. The classification of patients was one of the foundational pillars of moral treatment. Woodward believed "nothing is more important in an institution" than classification, stating that administrators should seek to "classify so that mutual good may be imparted, and so that no one shall associate with those particularly obnoxious to him" (Annual Report 1844: 89). In their designs, architects inscribed these classificatory schemes into the architectural arrangement of the asylum in the form of the Kirkbride plan, whose wards were segregated by gender, race, class, and disease type.

The premise of the therapeutic asylum hinged on its role as an embodiment and agent of moral treatment. In contrast to the harsh and coercive treatment of the mentally ill in the past, in the modern asylum the lunatic would "feel the benign influence of sympathy and compassion" and receive all "the benefits of pure air, occupation, and an agreeable mode of life" (Annual Report 1839: 5, 1844: 89). In practice, however, these ideals collided against the realities of overcrowding, limited budget, and the resistance of patients who actively contested the asylum's control over their minds and bodies. Ultimately the asylum itself, originally configured as the basis for moral treatment, formed the greatest obstacle to its implementation and progress. The materiality of the asylum as it was continuously inhabited, extended, and developed over decades served as a site for the inscription of meanings: a monument to its designers' "Follies" as well as a substrate for the exercise of patients' protest and autonomy. The asylum as "museum of madness" does not yield to one particular interpretation, but encompasses a multiplicity of functions and meanings, forming a complex and contradictory stratigraphy that speaks to the continuing ambiguity surrounding the legacy of the asylum.

THE PICTURESQUE ASYLUM

As envisioned by its creators, the practical function of the modern asylum as a therapeutic instrument would go hand in hand with its success as an aesthetic object. Writing in 1837, Dr. W. A. F. Browne stated that the ideal asylum should be "a spacious building resembling the palace of a peer" (Browne 1837: 226). In the United States, the architectural style first chosen to effect this resemblance was that of Gothic Revival. According to landscape architect Andrew Jackson Downing, the potency of the "bold and varied outlines" of Gothic Revival Style lay in their ability to "harmonize with picturesque scenery," such as the grounds he designed for the New Jersey State Lunatic Asylum and the New York State Asylum at Utica (Yanni 2007: 59). Although based on medieval European precedents, Gothic Style was mobilized by American architects as a "national architecture" believed to be suited to "our utilitarian age" and "matter-of-fact country," equally applicable to country estates, churches, and public edifices (Owen 1849: 67). As a European import that was adapted to American tastes and uses, Gothic architecture was a fitting emblem of moral treatment.

The recruitment of landscape architects such as Downing and Frederick Law Olmsted (responsible for the landscape design of the Buffalo State Asylum as well as New York City's Central Park) represented psychiatrists' investment in the Romantic approach to the built environment, which idealized Nature as the setting for transcendent emotional experiences (Picker 2003: 7). Asylums, parks, cemeteries, cities, and residences were all implicated in a Romantic ideology that linked health and the environment, aesthetics and therapeutics (Reiss 2008: 126). Natural beauty was believed to be inherently beneficial to health. Furthermore, the aesthetics of the salutary environment were not only visual but broadly experiential, engaging multiple senses. Landscapes were carefully choreographed to lead the body through a series of sensory encounters. These performative qualities were invested with the power to soothe the mind, nurture the body, and restore health. By shaping the natural environment into a site for control over patients' mental states, psychiatrists claimed a God-like mastery over both man and nature (Leone 2005: 241).

The recruitment of genteel landscape architects signaled superintendents' desire to civilize the asylum, locating it among a pantheon of structures—including churches, city halls, schools, and country estates—that indexed bourgeois gentility, pride in citizenship, and faith in human progress (Bushman 1993). Yet the asylum also belonged to another, darker architectural lineage: that of the stigmatized institutional forms of prisons, poorhouses, and workhouses. This mixed inheritance manifested in the material substrate of the asylum. Although psychiatric discourse emphasized the humane and gentle nature of moral treatment, the asylum as a physical object testifies to the reality that its interventions were largely coercive in nature. The palatial Gothic architecture chosen to ornament the asylum and enshrine its contribution to humanity existed in uneasy tension

with the barred windows, locked doors, and thick walls that were thought
to be necessary for its security. The filings for the construction of the first
hospital in 1833 contained 25 receipts for items related to security, including locks of various kinds, keys, grate bars, and expenditures related to the
construction of a special strong room for Howard Trask (table 1.1). In total,
administrators purchased over 210 locks, more than the number of patients
who were anticipated that first year. As the trustees of the Worcester State
Hospital wrote, the "architectural arrangement of a lunatic hospital is very
unlike that of a common dwelling or any other public institution. Walls,
partitions, windows, and doors must be much stronger" (Annual Report
1863: 30). The premise of moral treatment as a gentle intervention, which
worked by kindling the sparks of divine light within the patient, was belied
by the physicality of an asylum that was designed to subdue the protests of

**Table 1.1   Items Related to Security Purchased for the Worcester State Hospital, 1833.
Compiled from State Lunatic Hospital Filings, Massachusetts State Archives**

Item	Number	Cost	Vendor
Fitting room for Trask		$2.62	Merchant Tobey
Oak plank for Trask's room		$0.62	Merchant Tobey
Laying stone strong cells		$317.14	Ephraim Morse & William R. Wesson, Worcester
Grate bars	19.5	$1.00	W. A. Wheeler
Locks for w[ater?] closet	3	$1.62	Orlando Ware
Keys		$1.50	Orlando Ware
Key[?]		$0.13	Orlando Ware
8 in screwed dead locks	0.25 dozen	$2.75	Henry W. Miller
8 inch dead lock		$1.17	Henry W. Miller
¼ dozen Augers and 1 closet lock		$0.88	Henry W. Miller
½ dozen Wing's saw files & 2 stock locks		$0.90	Henry W. Miller
1 stock lock		$0.86	Henry W. Miller
4 inch dead lock		$0.33	Henry W. Miller
1 padlock, 1 iron kettle, wire		$0.36	Henry W. Miller
Dead locks	164	$328.00	Henry W. Miller
6 in fancy screwed dead locks	1 dozen	$5.00	Henry W. Miller
8 in fine dead lock		$1.00	Henry W. Miller
Long cupboard locks	2	$1.25	Henry W. Miller
Day's brass knobs for mortice locks	12 pair	$19.20	Henry W. Miller
4 inch long cupboard locks	2	$1.25	Henry W. Miller
8 inch dead lock		$1.00	Henry W. Miller
Closet locks	2	$0.50	Henry W. Miller
8 inch rim lock	1	$0.58	Henry W. Miller
Large bolts and keys and collars	103 lb	$10.30	Leonard Poole

resistant inmates. How effective was "the law of love" and "sympathy" if it was reliant on physical force (Annual Report 1833: 6)?

Describing the Worcester State Hospital in 1840, Woodward—known for his positive attitude, even among the unremitting optimists of the cult of curability—elides the coercive properties of the asylum in favor of eulogizing its most enlightened and civilized features. To him, the hospital was

> a fit emblem of the noble heart of the people, who generously founded and endowed it—spacious in its dimensions—as well ventilated, warmed, and supplied with pure water, and every other necessary and comfort of life, as any public institution in the whole world—with an infirmary for the sick, and a chapel for religious worship—with comfortable and airy apartments for the inmates, always kept clean and neat—with lofty open halls for their recreation and exercise, surrounded with ample grounds, and walks, and trees—placed on a high hill in full view of the magnificent amphitheatre of cultivated and ornamented highlands, which overlook and surround the beautiful town of Worcester—thus affording to the inmates of the hospital, a constant view of scenes well adapted to soothe, to delight and tranquilize their troubled minds. (Annual Report 1840: 4)

Woodward's description could have been pulled from contemporary Romantic literature that sentimentalized and sanctified nature as the antidote to the artifice of civilization. Yet the asylum was a decidedly *unnatural* entity—requiring the whole-scale remodeling of the environment, the introduction of foreign materials and new architectural techniques, and the careful orchestration of multiple sensory domains in order to produce its particular effects. The paradox of the Romantic view of nature cultivated by men like Olmsted, Downing, and Woodward was that it required such extensive manipulation—including a host of decidedly *unnatural* interventions—in order to meet cultural expectations for what was "natural" and aesthetically pleasing. The paradoxes and contradictions embedded in the foundation of asylum medicine would become increasingly apparent as the passage of time eroded the veneer of idealism surrounding the lunatic hospital.

"THE ENDURING ASYLUM"

The durability and monumentality of the hospital played an important role in the enactment of its illusions. The hospital was intended to embody strength and nobility, naturalizing its foundational paradigm and investing it with the character of a permanent and unimpeachable authority. Accordingly, the materials of the hospital were chosen not simply for their practicality but also for their contribution to this rhetorical statement. In the planning of the first hospital, the commissioners agreed that "no one would approve the use of a material less durable than brick or granite" (brick was ultimately chosen as the less expensive option) (The Commissioners 1832). The roof would be slated in order to provide "security against fire" and to reflect the "public character of the building, its solidity, and expected durability." When an addition was made in 1843, Woodward proudly reported that it was constructed of "solid masonry of stone and brick, which will stand for generations, a monument of [the benefactors'] well applied liberality" (Annual Report 1843: 8).

The use of "rough ashlar stone, quarried on the estate" to build the second hospital served to tie the building to its surroundings, in keeping with the Gothic impulse (articulated by Downing) to soften the boundary between built and "natural" environments, making the asylum seem as though it was an eternal feature rather than a recent imposition on the landscape. Like the Hudson River State Hospital—the first Kirkbride building constructed in what would come to be termed High Victorian Gothic Style—the second Worcester State Hospital featured "structural polychromy" in the form of brick belts, window casings, door jambs, and bay window projections, which "relieved the monotony that might arise in a building of this mass" (figure 1.1)

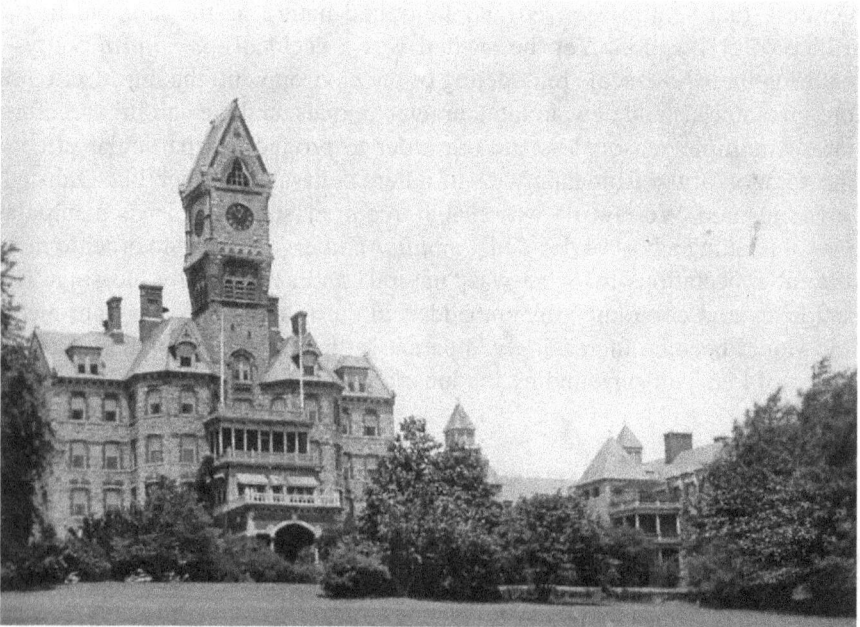

Figure 1.1   The Gothic Façade of the Second Worcester State Hospital, Shown Here in the 1920s. The cupolas were decorative elements used to disguise ventilation shafts. Courtesy of the Worcester Historical Museum.

(Yanni 2007: 113–114). A newspaper article announcing the opening of the hospital stated that "all the wall divisions are of brick, solid and of unusual thickness, and the whole structure is of the most substantial character" ("An important public structure completed" 1877). The windows were fitted with iron gratings and the gables were ornamented with iron finials. The roof was slate and the floors of hard pine (ibid.).

The "durational qualities" of the Worcester State Hospital and its counterparts had unintended consequences for their practical uses and ultimate legacy. While residential architects such as Gardner envisioned homes as "organic," dynamic entities, asylums were built to resist adaptability, retaining their original form and appearance. From an early period, psychiatrists realized that it would be difficult to adapt the asylum to meet its changing needs. Over time, these unwieldy and embarrassing structures came to represent monuments to the past that "intervene[d] in the present," preventing the development of the asylum building in accordance with changes in psychiatric thought (Hamilakis 2014: 123). Even when their use as hospitals ended, the stubborn materiality of asylums resisted adaptation. As Christopher Payne writes, the "very qualities that made [Kirkbride buildings] appealing in the first place"—namely their "size," "heavy construction," and "distinctive floor plan"—"have made them difficult to repurpose," a fact which has contributed to their widespread demolition by developers (Payne 2009: 13). Ironically, architects' drive to create structures that would last for an eternity ultimately rendered their creations disposable.

This physical durability was paralleled by the philosophical inflexibility of nineteenth-century psychiatry, which fiercely resisted changes to the design and construction of asylums. In 1851, the Association of Medical Superintendents of American Institutions for the Insane (AMSAII) established a set of standards known as the "26 rules" that its members would defend dogmatically for the rest of the century ("Report on the construction of hospitals for the insane" 1851: 79–80). According to the rules, an asylum should be located "in the country, not within less than two miles of a large town," yet be "easily accessible at all seasons." It should be "constructed of stone or brick," with "slate or metallic roofs," and be outfitted with "no less than 50 acres of land, devoted to gardens and pleasure grounds," which "should be surrounded by a substantial wall placed not to be unpleasantly visible from the building." The main structure should consist of a central building with wings, with each ward outfitted with a parlor, clothes room, bathroom, water closet, dining room, and dumbwaiter. The rule that would prove most controversial was that which limited the patient population to 250 ("preferably 200"). At their peak, many state hospitals would house well over a thousand patients; Worcester housed 2,400 in 1918 (Myerson 1980).[1]

AMSAII members' allegiance to the 26 rules reflected their belief that the principles of asylum construction—and, by extension, psychiatry—were universal and timeless because they were based on "natural" laws. As a result, asylum architects made little allowance for future changes and adaptations to their designs. Asylums continued to be constructed in much the same fashion throughout the nineteenth century, repudiating the lessons afforded by practical experience. With the advantages of hindsight—won by the hardships of living with their predecessors' mistakes—late nineteenth- and twentieth-century psychiatrists would acknowledge that the standards laid down in 1851 were nearsighted. As Albert Deutsch writes, "it was historical blindness to believe that the whole future could be fitted into the rigid framework of 26 rules" (Deutsch 1946: 211).

The failure to anticipate future needs had long-term effects on the Worcester State Hospital. Within fifteen years, nearly all of the therapeutic features Woodward had identified in the hospital of 1840 had been ravaged by time and overpopulation. The asylum's "spacious" interiors were crowded with people, its "comfortable and airy apartments" and "lofty open halls" strained past their capacity. The "amphitheatre of cultivated and ornamented highlands" that furnished the hospital with its therapeutic views had given way to urban development. Ventilation and plumbing systems that had been lauded as technologically advanced when they were installed in the 1830s were outmoded and deteriorating, because the wards were "so low studded," they could not be replaced (Annual Report 1856: 9). Likewise, walls of "unusual thickness" could not be easily shifted to rearrange the asylum's interior spaces. By the early 1850s, trustees recognized that the hospital was "obsolete" and believed it was "best to abandon it" (Annual Report 1854: 35). Nonetheless, budgetary restraints forestalled the construction of a replacement for more than twenty years.

ASYLUM HIERARCHIES

By the time the second hospital was built in the 1870s, public expectations for the modern asylum had changed. Partly due to the efficacy of psychiatrists in proselytizing moral treatment, patients and their families demanded "more extensive comforts, a better class of accommodations, improved style of architecture, and greater facilities for classification, treatment, recreation, and amusement" than the first generation of asylums provided (Annual Report 1866: 79). As a result of the decreased stigma surrounding institutionalization, middle- and upper-class families were increasingly willing to entrust their insane relatives to an asylum, creating a demand that drove the establishment of additional and increasingly specialized institutions. Some of these institutions, such as the Adams Nervine Asylum opened in 1880 outside of Boston, were dedicated to a private clientele suffering from "nervous" diseases (Adams Nervine Asylum 1880). In addition to an increased level of comfort and privacy, institutions such as Adams allowed middle- and upper-class patients to enjoy the advantages of institutionalized care while avoiding the stigmatizing label of insanity and the discomfort of association with the pauper insane.

The administrators of the Worcester State Hospital were keenly aware that the treatment of private patients not only furnished the asylum with much-needed income but also raised its public profile. They also knew that families who were able to pay for their relatives' care had more options than their lower-class counterparts, and could choose to transfer their relatives to a different hospital or keep them at home if they were displeased with the accommodations at Worcester.[2] This prerogative was exercised by the family of Jared Willson, who chose to have him transferred from an asylum in Litchfield, Connecticut, to the Connecticut Hospital for the Insane in Middletown in January 1889. Despite the fact that she had little hope of his recovery, Willson's mother was satisfied that Middletown was "the right place for him, as so much is done for comfort," citing the "extensive grounds that are finely cultivated" and variety of "entertainment[s]" (Willson 1889). Even families who relied on public support could exert a degree of agency in their relatives' treatment, such as Ella Tandberg, who appealed to Worcester trustee Rockwood Hoar to have her brother, a Civil War veteran suffering from neuralgia, placed in an institution that would provide more "pleasant surroundings" than his current residence in the Augusta State Hospital (Tandberg 1905).

At the same time that administrators were striving to meet the expectations of middle- and upper-class families, they were also faced with an increasing number of pauper patients. The hospital's patient population was further divided between those who were considered to be suffering from "acute" mental disease (which might resolve in a matter of weeks or months) and "chronic" cases that were considered largely hopeless. The conflicting demands of these distinct populations pulled administrators in opposite directions and challenged the identity and purpose of the hospital. While the State of New York responded to this dilemma by creating the Willard Asylum, a specialized institution for the chronically insane (Dwyer 1987), Worcester administrators were committed to maintaining an encyclopedic asylum that was (theoretically) capable of addressing the needs of any insane patient (with the exception of the criminally insane). The state hospital system was founded on the democratizing ideal of treatment for all citizens, regardless of wealth or social status; yet the asylum maintained a rigid hierarchy of patients. The experiences of patients in the asylum's upper tiers were dramatically different from those in the lowest, a fact that Elizabeth Packard learned firsthand when she was transferred from one of the "better" wards of the Jacksonville Asylum to one of the "worst" (Packard 1873).

Architectural arrangements quite literally set these hierarchies in stone. The earliest evidence of the use of architecture to marginalize certain patients at Worcester dates to 1833, when trustee W. B. Calhoun called for the construction of separate wards for "Africans" (Trustees 1833). By midcentury, the hospital had established dedicated wards for the Irish. Yet the patients who were most dramatically marginalized—at least in regard to spatial separation—were the so-called "violent" patients. Unlike their nonviolent counterparts, these individuals did not work, worship, or recreate with other patients, but were largely confined to the strong rooms, a set of unfurnished, prison-like cells that were designed with the primary objective of securing uncontrollable patients. Due to budgetary restraints, these cells were utilized long past the point of their obsolescence. Yet even when replacements were constructed in 1858, rendering the original strong rooms unnecessary, administrators did not demolish them, choosing instead to maintain them as "curious relic[s]" and "curiosities" (Annual Report 1858: 7). In 1863, the trustees wrote that the presence of the unoccupied strong rooms was "offensive and injurious, in reminding the patients of the harsher treatment of the insane in an olden time"—a curious statement given that the "olden time" in which the strong rooms had been used was only five years in the past (Annual Report 1862: 6).

The retention of outdated and dilapidated buildings alongside newer ones meant that the hospital functioned as an accretional structure or palimpsest. These accretions also included human beings. While the ideal patient entered the asylum, recovered, and was discharged in relatively quick succession (within six months to a year), many did not meet this expectation. Every year, a significant subset were not released and were given the status of "chronic" or "incurable." Although most of these patients were not violent and could be accommodated in a regular ward, their presence was inherently troublesome to administrators, who believed it shifted the character of the hospital from the curative to the custodial. According to the trustees, the Worcester State Hospital in 1875 contained six patients who had been confined there for more than 30 years, and eighteen who had been there more than 20 (Annual Report 1875: 32). Like the "Africans," the Irish, and the "violent," chronic patients were typically segregated: first in their own specialized wards, and later in both wards and farmhouses.

Beginning in 1895 at Worcester, "incurables" who were able to work were sent to the farmhouse on the edge of the property, and later to Hillside Farm in the neighboring town of Shrewsbury. Following the construction of the second Worcester State Hospital, its predecessor was quietly refashioned into an asylum for incurables known as the Asylum for the Chronic Insane[3] (later euphemistically renamed the "Summer Street Department"). Although administrators had complained for decades that the first hospital was danger- ously antiquated and dilapidated—the very complaints that had prompted the construction of its replacement in the first place—the accommodations were apparently acceptable for the lowest tier of the patient hierarchy, who were not provided with therapeutic treatment. A century after it was established as the embodiment of the promises of the new moral treatment, the Summer Street building had become a repository for its failures.

THE ASYLUM OF THE DEAD

The maintenance of chronic patients into old age inevitably raised the issue of the final deposition of their remains. Unlike many state institutions, Worcester did not initially allocate a space on its property for the burial of its dead. Instead, for more than a half century, patients who died in the hospital and had no relatives who were able to pay for their burials were interred in dedicated lots in Hope Cemetery (Annual Report 1851: 54). Although the cemetery itself was the property of the city of Worcester, responsibility for the maintenance of lots was charged to their respective owners. In 1862, the commissioners of Hope Cemetery complained about the failure of Worcester State Hospital administrators to uphold their agreement with the city:

> In the sale and conveyance of a large selected lot, some years since, to the Trustees of the State Lunatic Hospital in this city, it was the express understand- ing of the Commissioners with the Superintendent of that Institution, that the ground to be occupied should be inclosed [sic] by an appropriate and durable fence, and the inclosure [sic] so cultivated and adorned by the Grantees, as to render it an attractive and imposing spot in the Cemetery. Although several interments have since been made there, the Commissioners regret to notice, that no measures seem to have been taken for its improvement. (Commissioners of Hope Cemetery 1865: 56)

While dedicated to the dead, rural cemeteries such as Hope Cemetery were designed to be enjoyed by the living, functioning much like the asylum as places of healthful respite, genteel recreation, and communion with nature. And as in the case of the asylum, this genteel ideal existed in tension with the function of the cemetery as a depository for marginalized bodies. In order to minimize the intrusion of undesirables and reserve prime real estate for wealthier customers, city officials relegated "potter's fields" and institutional lots to the margins of the property. In striking its original agreement with the

Worcester State Hospital, the commissioners of Hope Cemetery formalized their expectations that the trustees would further modulate the impact of the mass grave of lunatics by bringing its lot into conformity with the standards of the Victorian rural cemetery.

While trustees' failure to supply the lot with a fence and "render it an attractive and imposing spot" may be partly attributed to their perpetually strained budget, they might have had other reasons to avoid drawing attention to the hospital's place in the cemetery. If the asylum stood as a monument to the promise of moral treatment, its cemetery lot represented a shrine to its failures that administrators might have preferred to ignore. Yet the accumulation of bodies exerted a material presence that couldn't be denied. Over the years, as its designated burial spaces reached their capacity, the hospital was forced to seek out new and increasingly marginal areas in which to locate their dead. In their 1872 report, the cemetery commissioners wrote that "the ground between Chestnut and Pine, and extending to Willow Avenue, which was grubbed and cleared in 1871, was carefully prepared for laying out early in spring" (Commissioners of Hope Cemetery 1872). Within this section, designated 41 and 42 on a contemporary map of the cemetery, "one hundred and eight lots were laid out" for the use of the Worcester State Hospital. By the late 1880s, the hospital was using section 19, in the far northeast corner of the cemetery, suggesting that the lot between Chestnut and Pine had been filled. Between 1888 and 1907, the records of the Hope Cemetery office indicate 331 burials from the hospital in section 19.[4] In 1916, administrators acknowledged that there was no longer any space in Hope Cemetery for the hospital's burials (Annual Report 1916: 8). In 1918, they designated a section of Hillside Farm in Shrewsbury as its new place of burial. The choice to locate the cemetery in Hillside, rather than on the hospital's main campus in Worcester, spoke to the continuing marginalization of chronic cases even after their deaths.

The "incurable" dead represented an even greater affront to the legitimacy of psychiatry than their living counterparts. While "chronic" patients may have been relegated to inferior wards and farmhouses and denied the benefits of the hospital's therapeutic program, the possibility of recovery—or at least improvement—existed as long as the patient was alive. Death foreclosed this possibility. The fact that a large number of the patients at the Worcester State Hospital would end their lives there, never escaping the confines of the institution even in death, dealt a punishing blow to the identity of the asylum as a curative institution. Furthermore, the failure of friends or family members to claim these patients' remains emphasized their doubly alienated status as lunatics and paupers, strangers in their own communities. Accordingly, the shame of the asylum's failed promise, as well as the stigma of insanity and poverty, likely both contributed to the decision to relegate patients' graves to marginal locations in Hope Cemetery and Hillside Farm, where today they can only be found by those who know where to look.

"MUSEUMS OF MADNESS"

With the dismantling of the cult of curability, hospitals that had once been viewed as symbols of progress and humanitarianism were fossilized into another type of icon entirely: monuments to the "Follies" of their creators, incapable of incorporating new developments in medicine and society (Bucknill 1876). In the latter half of the nineteenth century, asylums were disparaged as "hospital palaces" whose adornments formed only a thin veneer over their functional inadequacies. The same aesthetic qualities that had once made the asylum "a fit emblem of the noble heart of the people" came to be associated with failure and retroversion. According to William Godding, by 1890 the first asylums were perceived as sites of "oppressive splendor," consisting of "vast hall spaces lined with settees, stately gothic, medieval in their discomfort, drafty corridors, blank white walls, polished floors coldly beautiful in their cleanliness that suggest a skating rink" (Godding 1890: 5).

This shift in the perception of the asylum placed psychiatrists on the defensive. "What are called palatial buildings have been a great advantage to the world," Orpheus Everts wrote in the *American Journal of Insanity.* "It is the difference between a hospital and a bedlam" (Everts 1878: 159). Notably, this distinction hinged on the buildings themselves, rather than the program of treatment carried on within their walls. Facing the challenge of public opinion as well as criticism from within the discipline, psychiatrists doubled down on the Edifice Complex. "We should ask ourselves whether, with better-planned hospitals, we may not be able to do better work," John B. Chapin wrote in the *American Journal of Insanity* in 1892. "Suitable plans are as essential to the best results of hospital work as improved machinery is to the manufacturer" (Chapin 1892: 188). If the asylum had not yielded the expected number of cures, then it must be due to a fault in its architectural design. New designs were therefore pursued as the only solution.

As a model for these designs, psychiatrists looked to the general hospital, which in the post-Civil War era enjoyed a rising public profile. In doing so, administrators hoped both to augment the asylum's therapeutic powers and soften its stigmatized features. In the 1899 annual report, trustees boasted that a visitor to one of Worcester's new wards "sees almost nothing to remind him that he is in an insane hospital, and might easily persuade himself that he was visiting one of the newest and best wards of Roosevelt, or the Mass[achusetts] General Hospital" (Annual Report 1899: 6). Yet most of these changes were limited in scope; only a small number of patients occupied the new wards, while the majority was relegated to the antiquated spaces of the main Kirkbride complex. When psychiatrists attempted to alter their treatment programs to keep pace with changes in psychiatric doctrine, they continued to collide against the stubborn materiality of the asylum. "For more than twenty years I have been trying to 'individualize treatment,'" Charles Bancroft complained—referencing the call for psychiatrists to cater to the needs of the individual patient—"but at most points have been headed off by brick and mortar walls" (Bancroft 1888: 128). Once the premiere symbol and instrument of psychiatry, the asylum had become the biggest impediment to its progress.

Psychiatrists were able to learn from some of the mistakes of their predecessors. J. P. Bancroft wrote that "[t]he building ought to represent at once the largest knowledge and practical experience of the alienist physician, reduced to forms of convenience and grace by the architect" (Bancroft 1889: 386). Yet he conceded that he "would now regard it unwise to make any general declaration of principles" regarding asylum architecture. "Any propositions we might adopt are but announcements of opinions held today, which 20 years hence may come to be regarded as inapplicable platitudes"—precisely what had happened to the 26 rules that AMSAII had established in 1851. Yet despite these insights, asylum architects continued to fall into the same traps that snared their predecessors. While the second Worcester State Hospital was being built, administrators realized that the building would be insufficient for the number of patients who were waiting to fill it—meaning that the hospital had been rendered obsolete before it was even finished. Architects scrambled to alter their plans in the midst of construction, raising the capacity of hospital to 400 patients (well above AMSAII's recommended limit of 250). Within ten years, that capacity was further increased to 600 by appropriating specialized rooms for dormitories (Annual Report 1892: 14). This was also a violation of AMSAII's rules, which stipulated that each ward should be equipped with its own parlor, corridor, clothes room, and dining room. In time, most of these spaces—as well as hallways and stairwells—would be colonized by patient beds. This was the unsavory bargain struck by the asylum of the late nineteenth century: to accept an ever greater number of patients at the expense of the resources that offered them the best chance of recovery.

Treasurers' reports further testify to the unpleasant arithmetic used to maintain a basic quality of life for the hospital's patients at the expense of the therapeutic ideal. These reports, which were intended to keep the public apprised to how the hospital was spending taxpayer funds, itemize the hospital's expenditures by categories, including "improvements and repairs," "furniture, crockery, & bedding," "provisions and groceries," "fuel & lights," and "clothing, linen, &c." With the increasing size of the hospital and the inflation of currency over time, the hospital's expenditures increased radically (figure 1.2). Yet the rate of increase differed substantially between

Expenditures of the Worcester State Hospital, 1833-1940

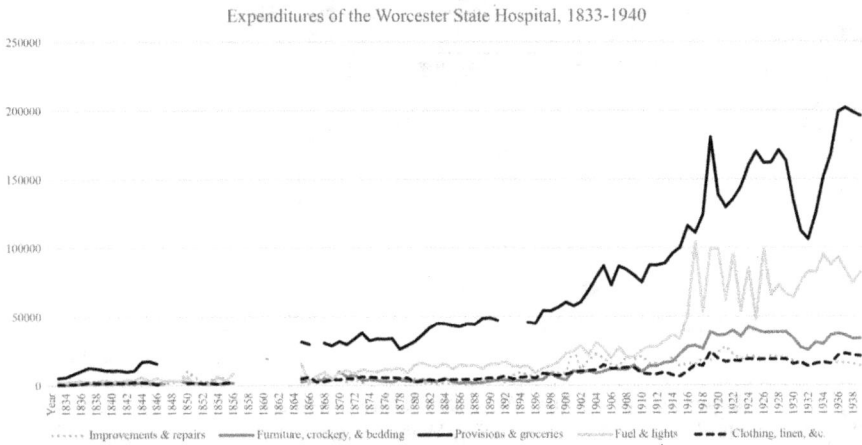

Figure 1.2 Expenditures of the Worcester State Hospital, 1833–1940. Gaps indicate years for which this data was not enumerated in the treasurer's report. Created by the author.

categories. "Provisions and groceries"—the goods needed to maintain the barest level of existence – increased the most dramatically, particularly after 1900, perhaps reflecting the reverberations of the 1902 nurses' strike, during which a public spotlight was placed upon the allegedly low quality of food at the hospital (see chapter 5). "Fuel & lights"—necessary to heat and illuminate the increasingly vast spaces of the hospital, also increased at a rapid pace, particularly after the electrification of the hospital in 1905. In contrast, expenditures for "improvements & repairs," "furniture, crockery & bedding," and "clothing, linen, &c." increased more slowly.

Similarly, while the salaries and wages paid by the hospital to its employees kept pace with inflation, and increased rapidly after 1915, the allocation made for improvements & repairs forms virtually a flat line (figure 1.3). A closer analysis of the proportion of the budget allocated to the maintenance of the hospital reveals distinct trends (figure 1.4). In the first two decades of the hospital, this allocation represented a significant part of the hospital budget, ranging from 2 to 15%. This percentage decreased in the 1870s and 1880s, most likely due to the construction of the second Worcester State Hospital, replacing its dilapidated predecessor. After ten years of wear and tear, however, expenditures for maintenance once again began to rise, reaching a high point of 7% in 1900, only to drop off quickly in the twentieth century.

The decreased expenditures allocated to maintenance were reflected in the physical decay of the hospital. By 1906, the thirty-year-old institution was considered "antiquated" (Annual Report 1906: 12). Its deterioration not only

Expenditures of the Worcester State Hospital, 1833-1940

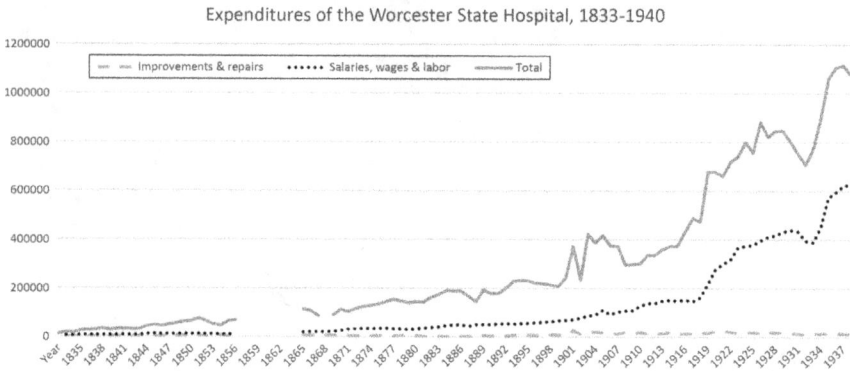

Figure 1.3 **Expenditures of the Worcester State Hospital, 1833–1940, Comparing "Improvements & Repairs" and "Salaries, Wages & Labor" against Total Expenditures.** Created by the author.

Percentage of funds spent on improvements & repairs, 1833-1940

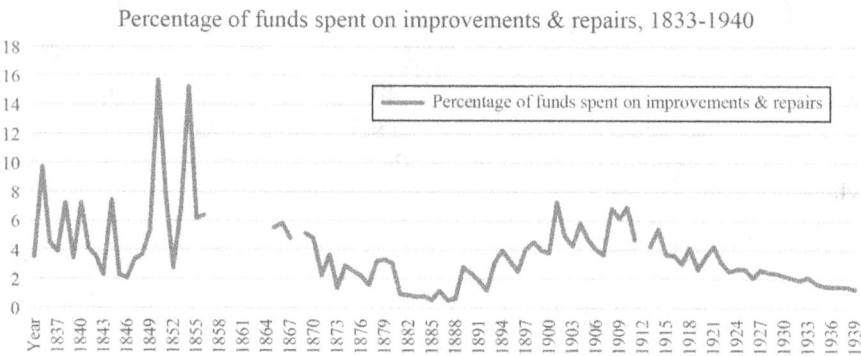

Figure 1.4 **Percentage of Funds Spent on Improvements and Repairs, 1833–1940.** Created by the author.

compromised its therapeutic efficacy but also posed a direct threat to patients' lives. Ironically, buildings that had been constructed as monumental and durational structures demonstrated a remarkable tendency to spontaneously self-destruct, and when they did, the results were often tragic. In 1888, the traumatized superintendent of the Cleveland Asylum, Jamin Strong, wrote to Pliny Earle describing a series of deadly fires in his institution. Like the Worcester State Hospital, the Cleveland Asylum consisted of a patchwork of different structures, many of which were dangerously outmoded. The continued utilization of the asylum's oldest structures, which Strong described as "combustible as a tinder box," resulted in a series of fires that claimed the lives of six patients and one nurse (Strong 1888). In the place of the destroyed buildings, Strong reported that "excellent, fire-proof structures, isolated from the Asylum buildings proper" were now under construction. Despite efforts to fireproof the complex, the Worcester State Hospital would ultimately fall victim to the same fate in 1933, when a fire consumed part of the roof, and in 1991, when a fire consumed the (then unoccupied) Kirkbride complex, leaving most of the building gutted.

ENDING THE EDIFICE COMPLEX

Pliny Earle was one of the first psychiatrists to openly challenge the premise and results of the cult of curability, and by extension, the Edifice Complex. In 1879, he wrote that "the question of the best system of managing the insane is more unsolved than 40 years ago; then it was apparently solved simply by construction of hospitals; now it has become a mystery by the inadequacy of hospitals to accomplish the desired end" (Earle 1879: 13). Within the next few decades, additional voices joined in, arguing that hospital administrators should redirect their focus away from the architecture and physical logistics of the asylum and toward research projects. "It has been a cause of reproach to the lunatic hospitals of Massachusetts," wrote the trustees of the Worcester State Hospital in 1895, "as well as to those of other States, that they are little more than enormous boarding-houses for the care of the insane" (Annual Report 1895: 6). In response, they hired pathologist Adolf Meyer, who established a laboratory at Worcester to research the causes of and treatment for mental diseases. Over the next decades, administrators would push for the refashioning of the asylum as a center for scientific research, training, and experimentation. By 1897, they boasted that "Meyer's work in the hospital and laboratory is placing us in the front ranks of like institutions in the country" (Annual Report 1897: 6).

This shift in the identity of the institution was couched in terms of the "advancement of medical and pathological science," in contrast to the former myopic focus on the materiality of the asylum and the everyday minutiae of its administration. But the prioritizing of research resulted in a different type of objectification: the transformation of patients into "material" for study. The classification of patients no longer functioned as a means of cure, but instead as a strategy for ordering the different varieties of insanity in the same way that a collector might arrange natural specimens. Within this system, the value of the patient's life was a function of its contribution to research and training, and the hospital was reconceptualized as a site for the production of scientific knowledge, rather than cure. In 1895, the trustees expressed their regrets "that a vast amount of valuable material for scientific observation"— that is, patients—had "been wasted" prior to the establishment of Meyer's laboratory (Annual Report 1895: 6).

"MATERIAL SIGNATURES"

In addition to its ideological function, the solidity of the asylum was also intended to resist patients' destructive tendencies. Yet the asylum was never fully invulnerable to the interventions of patients, whose continuous use of and resistance against the material substrate of the buildings they inhabited formed one of the foremost points of contact between individual and institution, design, and practice. Acts of destruction were not merely expressions of insanity but also of protest, conducted through the medium of the asylum itself. Clifford Beers broke the glass ceiling lamp in his cell as a means of provoking the attendants, whom he viewed as criminally negligent in their duties (Beers 1913: 57). Afterward, he used the pieces of the lamp to carve the message into the door of his cell: "God bless our Home, which is Hell." In inscribing their commentaries directly onto the object of their protest, patients such as Beers staked a claim to define the nature of the building according to their own perceptions and experiences, which often stood dramatically at odds with the image of the asylum conjured by its administrators. Beers's description of the asylum as a "Home" that is really "Hell" makes a mockery of administrators' attempts to domesticate the institution. In tracing these "material signatures" of confinement into the asylum, patients appropriated its materiality for their own purposes, remaking the asylum into a living text for the inscription of their agency (Casella 2009: 31).

Many patients took advantage of vulnerabilities in the material fabric of the Worcester State Hospital in order to stage their escapes, the ultimate act of protest against confinement. In 1834, trustee Thomas Kinnicutt reported that a patient named Mr. Coolidge "escaped from one of the cells in the Lodge, by loosening the bricks with a nail or some other small instrument, and making an aperture large enough for his body to pass." Kinnicutt added that this incident was Coolidge's "second escape from the same building effected on account of its want of strength" (Trustees' Notes 1834). Apparently, the cells in the Lodge—also known as the "strong rooms" and constructed out of "hard burnt bricks laid in water cement" (Annual Report 1849: 6)—were not as strong as their name suggested, perhaps reflecting the budgetary and time constraints under which they were constructed. Typically, patients' desire to escape confinement was viewed by psychiatrists as a symptom of insanity, while acceptance of treatment and willingness to submit to asylum discipline was indicative of recovery. However, trustees' reports provide ample documentation of the reasons why anyone, insane or not, would want to escape the strong rooms (see chapter 3).

Psychiatrists viewed acts of defiance against the asylum building and its furnishings as threatening both to the practical and ideological functioning of the asylum. In 1879 A. P. Reid, superintendent of the Nova Scotia Hospital for the Insane, complained in a letter to Pliny Earle about the difficulty of obtaining "'chambers' and 'spittoons' in the violent wards that will not break and cannot be used as weapons of offense, and that are not heavy" (Reid 1879). Earle had his own strategy for combating patient destruction: holding them financially responsible. A year earlier, he had received an angry letter from Clinton D. Miner protesting the bill he had received for clothes and a chamber pot that he had allegedly destroyed while confined to the Northampton State Hospital (Miner 1878). In a note appended to the letter, Earle itemized Miner's acts of destruction, accusing him of tearing a pair of socks and throwing another pair down a ventilator, tearing three shirts, and destroying a bedstead. In his reply to Miner, Earle wrote that "[w]e are not in the habit of charging things to persons that we do not furnish to them; or of charging damages unless those damages are done," and suggested that Miner could not remember his acts of destruction because he had been insane at the time (Earle 1878). Earle had been recruited as superintendent of the Northampton State Hospital primarily to take control of the asylum's finances; the relentless pursuit of reimbursement from Miner is emblematic of the strict and economical approach upon which Earle built his reputation. Having contributed to the destruction of the "cult of curability," Earle viewed the primary role of the asylum not as a therapeutic instrument but as a business.

CLOTHING

In addition to the building, its environment, and its furnishings, administrators also considered the influence that clothing exerted over patients' physical and mental states. As the primary interface between the self and the outside world, clothing formed a microarchitecture of the body, playing a key role in the modulation of the senses. Depending on the nature of the sensory experiences that it enabled or inhibited, clothing could have either healthful or pernicious effects. The dichotomy between health and pathology neatly mapped onto the dyad between nature and artifice, enabling psychiatrists to assume the role of sartorial police. They asserted that "healthful" clothing shielded the body against the elements and properly regulated temperature served the body's natural functions; conversely, clothing that was designed primarily to adorn the body and contort it into unnatural shapes, sacrificing well-being for the sake of the latest fashions, was "artificial" and thus unhealthy. Bourgeois morality formed an implicit role in structuring these oppositions, pinning what was healthful to what was good, and what was artificial and unhealthy to the sins of pride and vanity.

Woodward wrote extensively on the harmful effects of fashionable clothing. He disparaged rubber shoes, which he believed were insufficient to warm
the feet. Like J. R. Black, Woodward believed that "nearly all diseases are
the result of exposure to cold" (Black 1873). The pernicious effects of cold
feet in particular were so radical that most "invalids, affected by diseases of
the head, or of the nervous system," could be restored to health simply by
"restoring warmth to these extremities" (Woodward n.d.). On the other hand,
the wearing of furs and other warm clothing could heat the body excessively,
which Woodward believed had particularly negative consequences for men,
as "effeminate habits are established by too great care in regard to clothing
and warmth." Tight collars and cravats cut off circulation, leading to "accumulation of blood upon the brain," which could result in syncope and even
"sudden death" (ibid.). While couched in medical language, such arguments
betray the influence of social discourses governing respectability, morality,
and gender. To Woodward, vanity was not simply a sin against God, but also
a crime against nature. For a man to be "effeminate" was not only a social
transgression that threatened concepts of masculinity but also evidence of
aberrant physiology.

Despite their disparagement of the "pernicious" effects of fashion, psychiatrists did acknowledge the importance of the social function of clothing
and its role in the rehabilitation of the insane. For asylum patients, clothing
provided much-needed social and moral structure. "In regulating the dress
of the insane, as in every regulation for them, we must consider not only its
first and indispensable uses, but its effects upon the mind," Conolly wrote
(Conolly 1847: 52). Neglect of dress was a noted symptom of insanity, and
inevitably went along with "degradation" and loss of "self-respect." In his
annual reports, Woodward described the links between clothing and patients'
behavior, believing that certain styles of dress held the capacity to form mental character. "If [a patient] is neatly and comfortably clad," he wrote, "like
those whom he meets, he feels that he is as good as others, respects himself
as they appear to respect him, and is careful to do nothing by which he shall
'lose caste.' If his garments are tattered and dirty, he will tear them off or soil
them more, if neat and tidy, he will preserve them with care and even feel
proud of them" (Annual Report 1839: 96).

In emphasizing the importance of dress, Conolly and Woodward identified
the social persona of the insane as crucial to health and identity, viewing it
as a buttress against which the patient could avoid giving way to the hall-
marks of "advanced and incurable forms of disorder" (Conolly 1847: 64).
The ability to maintain an identity congruent with that of the outside world
maintained the hope that the severance of social linkages was only temporary, and that one's place in society might someday be restored. In this way,
psychiatrists sought to counter the dehumanizing effects that were suffered

archetypally by the lunatic who was reduced to rags or nakedness. Yet in doing so, these psychiatrists also reified social norms as natural and medically justified. Respectability in appearance—and particularly the kind which encoded one's social status—functioned as an index of mental health, with "negligence or peculiarity of dress" pathologized as a symptom of insanity (ibid.: 61-4). Conversely, the ability to maintain a respectable appearance, appropriate to status, occasion, and season, was naturalized. Believing that the enclosure of the body within a normative and familiar mode of dress would encourage the adoption of the associated habits and frame of mind, Conolly wrote that patients should wear the types of clothes they had worn before the onset of illness, tailored to their individual character and to their "station" in life. For this reason, administrators should carefully police inmates' dress, ensuring that proper clothing was worn while avoiding the stigmatizing attire of institutionalization. Browne cautioned that "uniformity of costume . . . reminds one of the workhouse, prison, and galley-slave" (Browne 1837: 188). Photographs from the Worcester State Hospital from the nineteenth and early twentieth centuries suggest that patients typically did not wear uniforms, with the exception of certain activities, such as outdoor exercise (figures 1.5 and 1.6).

Uniforms assumed a different meaning when they were offered to asylum attendants, for whom they served an "honorific" rather than "stigmatic" function (Hamlett 2013: 98). Superintendents reported that "where uniforms have been introduced the *espirit de corps* of the attendants has been increased and the service has assumed new importance" ("Uniforming attendants" 1886: 127–128). Uniforms served to "elevate the standard" and "increase the permanency of asylum service." Perhaps most importantly from the attendants' perspective, uniforms served to distinguish them from patients. As will be discussed in chapter 3, much of the conflict between patients and attendants may be traced to their uncomfortable proximity in social status. Uniforms served to elevate their wearers above the level of pauper lunatics and secure their status as professionals. Furthermore, uniforms enabled third parties to distinguish staff from patients, a task that was always more difficult than expected. In asylums where both patients and staff wore street clothes, "keys were the only true guarantee of non-patient status" (Callaway 2007: 26).

Clothing and Patient Protest

Just as clothing served as a site for the performance of institutional and social identities, it could also serve as the site of their contestation or undoing. Among the forms of patient misconduct, the removal of or refusal to wear clothing was viewed by administrators as one of the most troubling and threatening to institutional order. Nakedness represented a repudiation

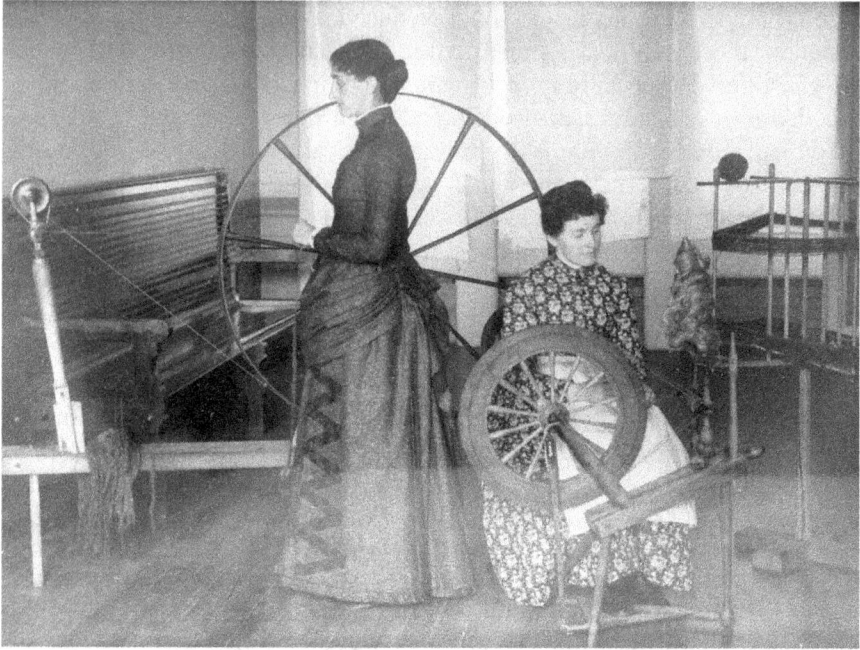

Figure 1.5 Patients Spinning at the Worcester State Hospital, circa 1870s-1880s. While the clothing and behavior of the two women would have passed without notice in a domestic setting, the presence of the distinctive hard, straight-backed settee in the background marks the space as institutional. Courtesy of the Worcester Historical Museum.

of both social norms and the organized regime of hospital management, as well as a threat to health. When faced with these challenges, administrators sacrificed the pursuit of normality in patient dress for the practicalities of "secure" clothing. The durability of these items paralleled that of the asylum itself. "Those who tear clothing must have it of ticking, or some other strong material," wrote Conolly, while "those who undress themselves must have clothes fastened by small locks instead of buttons" (Conolly 1847: 92). While articulated as necessary for patient safety, such "secure clothing" could also be "utilized as stigmatic punishment" (Wynter 2010: 51), serving to strip the patient not only of freedom but also of respectability. At the Worcester State Hospital, this was sometimes a losing battle. W. B. Calhoun, a trustee reporting on the conditions of the hospital in the winter of 1834, suggested that the heat in the strong rooms was maintained at such a level to provide comfort to "patients [who] divest themselves of their clothing" (Trustees 1834).

The process whereby patients were dressed for the asylum, "transform[ing] lunatics into looked-after patients," was heavily ritualized and freighted

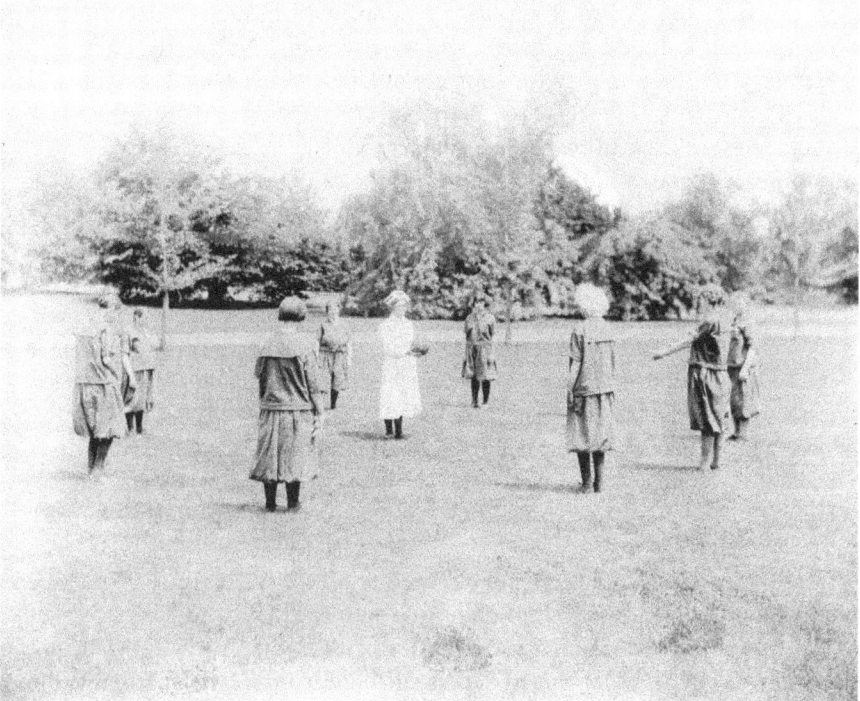

Figure 1.6   A Scene of Recreation at the Worcester State Hospital Showing Patients Wearing the Same Athletic Outfit (Undated; Early Twentieth Century). Courtesy of the Worcester Historical Museum.

with symbolic meaning (Wynter 2010: 45). The commissioners who super-intended the construction of the first Worcester State Hospital resolved that the lunatics brought to the new asylum from their makeshift lodgings in the towns of Massachusetts should

> be put into a state of perfect bodily cleanliness before removed, and to clothe them all in an entire new dress,* on their being taken from their respective places of confinement, in order that this unfortunate class of our fellow beings may realize every benefit which can be derived from a favorable change in their physical sensations, combined with a change of residence, of regiment, and of moral treatment. (The Commissioners 1833)

The asterisk indicated that this dress "should be of a mixed color or Oxford grey satinet, and that each patient should come provided with a change of linen, and of socks, and a pair of shoes." These presumably would be provided by the patients' respective towns, which in the first decades of the asylum were financially responsible for the care and treatment of their insane.

In practice, the desire to furnish patients with attractive and functional clothing often collided against budgetary restraints. Nelly Bly reported the inadequacy of clothing provided for her at Blackwell's Island Asylum:

> One underskirt made of coarse dark cotton goods and a cheap white calico dress with a black spot on it. I tied the strings of the skirt around me and put on the little dress. It was made, as are all those worn by the patients, into a straight tight waist sewed on to a straight skirt. As I buttoned the waist I noticed the underskirt was about six inches longer than the upper, and for a moment I sat down on the bed and laughed at my own appearance. No woman ever longed for a mirror more than I did at that moment. My hair, all matted and wet from the night previous, was pulled and jerked, and, after expostulating to no avail, I set my teeth and endured the pain. They refused to give me my hairpins, and my hair was arranged in one plait and tied with a red cotton rag. I asked that we be given additional clothing, at least as much as custom says women shall wear, but they told me to shut up; that we had as much as they intended to give us. (Bly 1887)

In this way, institutional clothing served to efface the identity of the wearer and to dehumanize him or her. Echoing Woodward, Clifford Beers wrote that clothes "have a sobering and civilizing effect" (Beers 1913: 84). During his confinement to the violent ward, Beers suffered from a lack of suitable clothing, which worsened his mental state and behavior. Once he was "provided with presentable outer garments [his] conduct rapidly improved." Beers's account suggests the ways in which the asylum's dominion over clothing as the source for respectability, identity, and basic comfort could be weaponized against patients in order to control their behavior. At the Worcester State Hospital, only the "better classes" of patients were allowed to keep "trunks in their own rooms" with access to their own "clothing, books, and work" (Annual Report 1839: 89). The personal items belonging to "excited" patients were held and closely policed by attendants. Under Conolly's instruction, the clothing of patients in the violent wards at Hanwell was removed from their bedrooms at night in order to prevent the use of the material for self-harm or escape (Conolly 1847: 99).

FURNISHINGS

Like clothing, the furnishings of the asylum could function as a substrate for the performance of both sanity and madness. Echoing Woodward's statements about clothing, superintendent F. Needham described the furnishings of the asylum as holding agentive powers, capable of influencing patients' mental states and of bringing their behavior in line with civilized norms.

It is certain that whereas delicate surroundings conduce to delicate ways and movements, coarse furniture contributes to coarse habits. A man smokes his pipe and spits upon the earthen floor, but something would prevent him doing either in a carpeted drawing room. What is true in this respect of insane persons is no less true of those who are deprived of reason. The insane man is too often a sane man decivilized, and to him the various processes of civilization have again to be applied. (Edgington 2007: 99)

W. F. Evans expressed similar ideas in *Mental Medicine* (1872). Quoting Longfellow, he stated that "all houses are haunted houses." The "influence of inanimate objects" derives from the "material effluvia" and "psychical emanations" that they produce (Evans 1872: 83). This influence was exaggerated in the insane, whose sensory perceptions were believed to be heightened by their disease. Accordingly, the "sight of some trivial object— a door, a paper-hanging, or a piece of furniture" was capable of exciting "a train of uncomfortable reflections" (Ray 1863: 323). It is for this reason that the furnishings of the patient's own home were thought to be inappropriate for the period of his recovery; they should be replaced by the furnishings of the asylum, which were neutralized of meaning and devoid of historical associations.

According to Conolly, the rooms of the insane should be simply but tastefully furnished, with a "light cast-iron bedstead," "a little carpet or coir matting, chair or small bench" (Conolly 1847: 20). A great deal of attention should be devoted to "curable patients," who could be lured from the isolation of their rooms by wards fitted with "a better style of furniture," with "an open fire in winter, books, pictures, plants, &c." (Ray 1846). In a letter written to Hugh Bell in 1845, Woodward itemized the furnishings of a standard patient's room at the Worcester State Hospital: a "single bed, mattress, pillow, bedstead, blankets, counterpane, [and] sheets . . . table, chairs, glass, [and] 2 yards of carpet," which were valued at a total of $25 (Woodward 1845). Attendants' rooms were furnished identically, but were given a double bed and higher quality carpet, for a total value of $50. While potentially curable patients may have been prioritized in the allotment of tasteful furnishings in the asylum, even the "incurable insane" could be positively influenced by "taste and tidiness in the decoration of the ward," according to an article in the *American Journal of Insanity:* "Pleasantly tinted walls, neat floors, tasty curtains, comfortable furniture, and bright rugs produce a marvelous effect" ("The favorable modification . . . " 1895). Conolly noted that items such as a "washing stand, box, looking glass, [and] small chest of drawers" were "most necessary for the incurable for whom the asylum is their only home" (Conolly 1847: 22).

In practice, however, patient accommodations—particularly for those patients who were considered incurable or violent—were not always so well appointed. According to the trustees of the Worcester State Hospital, the maintenance of a home-like interior was undermined by the considerations of durability and expense, "on account of damage/destruction from [patients'] violence and mischief" (Annual Report 1837: 13). Certain items were selectively eliminated from patients' surroundings. Depending on an individual patient's behavior, he or she might be housed in a ward with relatively normal furnishings, or—if he or she were violent or ill-behaved—secluded in an unfurnished and windowless room. In the violent ward, Clifford Beers wrote that "the walls and floor were bare, and there was no furniture" (Beers 1913: 70). In the insane ward of Bellevue Hospital, Nellie Bly reported that "several still-looking benches and a number of willow chairs were the only articles of furniture" (Bly 1887). This variability in the furnishings of apartments pinned patient behavior and its associated mental state to the material support of their surroundings, forming subsidiary spheres of experience within the larger architecture of the asylum. The material world served as a structure for organizing—and thereby disciplining—patients.

Receipts from purchases made for the initial construction of the Worcester State Hospital in 1833 reveal the variety of furnishings used in the institution and the potential for their use in differentiation between subsets of its population (table 1.2). Given the potential for patients' "violence and mischief," it is unlikely that the two looking glasses purchased for $12 from the John Doggett Looking Glass & Carpet Warehouse in Boston were intended to adorn the walls of the wards. John Doggett was known for his refined and elegant looking glasses, picture frames, and furniture "in the classical taste favored by Boston's elite" (Nylander 2016). Accordingly, these mirrors were most likely intended for the superintendent's quarters or for the public spaces of the building used for entertaining visitors.

Administrators also purchased three looking glasses from George T. Rice & Co. for a total of $1.13. While these mirrors may have been intended to adorn the walls of the "better" wards—which included genteel furnishings such as framed pictures and pianofortes—the discrepancy between the number of mirrors (a total of five in the hospital's initial purchases) and the hospital population suggests that only a minority would have enjoyed access to these items. Other categories of items purchased for the hospital indicate similar discrepancies. High-quality goods were purchased in small quantities, presumably to be reserved for the hospital's staff, visitors, and possibly by private and well-behaved patients. These goods include three couches purchased from Samuel Beal & Sons, valued at $32, $32, and $25, respectively; a Madison case of drawers valued at $14; a counting house desk for $14; two mahogany tables for $9.00 and $8.00, respectively; two "French bedsteads" for $8.50; and two bureaus for $14 each. In contrast, low-quality, inexpensive goods were purchased in large quantities, presumably for the

Table 1.2 Furnishings Purchased for the Worcester State Hospital, 1833. Compiled from State Lunatic Hospital Filings, Massachusetts State Archives

Item	Number	Price	Vendor
Imitation maple chairs	18	$19.50	Miller & Wood, Worcester
Dark common chairs	24	$12.00	Miller & Wood, Worcester
Copper finished fancy chairs	4	$4.00	Miller & Wood, Worcester
Dark fancy chairs	12	$12.00	Miller & Wood, Worcester
Large rocking chairs	2	$6.00	Miller & Wood, Worcester
Dark fancy top chairs	12	$5.00	Miller & Wood, Worcester
Small rocking chairs	2	$2.50	Miller & Wood, Worcester
Fine carpeting	30 yds	$30.00	Livermore & Kendall, Boston
Carpeting	22 yds	$3.13	William H. Swan
Hearth rugs	2	$9.00	William H. Swan
Bedsteads	12	$42	Samuel Beal & Sons, Worcester
Small lamps	2	$0.67	Rice & Sweetser
Large lamps	2	$1.17	Rice & Sweetser
Couch	1	$32	Samuel Beal & Sons, Worcester
Couch	1	$32	Samuel Beal & Sons, Worcester
Couch	1	$25	Samuel Beal & Sons, Worcester
Bureau	1	$14	Samuel Beal & Sons, Worcester
Bureau	1	$14	Samuel Beal & Sons, Worcester
Piland[?] tables	1	$18.00	Samuel Beal & Sons, Worcester
Raymond chairs	12	$10	Samuel Beal & Sons, Worcester
Fine carpeting		$78.20	Livermore & Kendall, Boston
Rugs	2	$0.80	Benjamin Leeds, Boston
Looking glasses	2	$12.00	John Doggett Looking Glass & Carpet Warehouse, Boston
4 by 5 ft mahogany table		$9.00	Lansford Wood & Co., Worcester
4 ft mahogany table		$8.00	Lansford Wood & Co., Worcester
Light wash stands	2	$3.33	Lansford Wood & Co., Worcester
Dark wash stands	3	$3.00	Lansford Wood & Co., Worcester
Dark dress table	1	$1.75	Lansford Wood & Co., Worcester
Madison Case of Drawers	1	$14.00	Lansford Wood & Co., Worcester
Counting House Desk	1	$14.00	Lansford Wood & Co., Worcester
4.5 ft table with drawer	1	$7.00	Lansford Wood & Co., Worcester
Cherry table		$3.00	Lansford Wood & Co., Worcester
4 ft cherry table		$6.50	Lansford Wood & Co., Worcester
French bedsteads	2	$8.50	Lansford Wood & Co., Worcester
Bed cords	2	$1.00	Lansford Wood & Co., Worcester
Single bedstead		$3.00	Lansford Wood & Co., Worcester
Window blinds	40 pr	$120.00	Lowes Brown
Blinds for two Venetian windows		$4.50	Lowes Brown
Hair mattresses	10	$37.50	John G. Flagg, Boston
Hair mattresses	20	$74.40	John G. Flagg, Boston
Hair mattresses	50	$187.50	John G. Flagg, Boston

(Continued)

Table 1.2 Furnishings Purchased for the Worcester State Hospital, 1833. Compiled from State Lunatic Hospital Filings, Massachusetts State Archives (Continued)

Item	Number	Price	Vendor
Hair mattresses, double	8	$56.00	John G. Flagg, Boston
Hair mattresses, single	20	$75.00	John G. Flagg, Boston
Bedstead & cord		$4.46	Elbridge G. Partridge, Worcester
Bedsteads	8	$28.00	Elbridge G. Partridge, Worcester
Bedsteads	15	$45.00	Stephen Bellows, Worcester
Plain small lamps	1 pair	$0.33	Rice & Sweetser
Five looking glasses and one bed cord		$2.38	George T. Rice & Co.
Looking glasses	3	$1.13	George T. Rice & Co.
Bedsteads for hospital patients	50	$150	Robert G. Taft
Bedsteads	20	$65.00	Stephen Bellows
Bedsteads	10	$32.50	Stephen Bellows
Bed lamps	1 dozen	$1.[cut off]	George T. Rice & Co., Worcester
Dish lamps	½ dozen	$1.00	George T. Rice & Co., Worcester
Entry lamp		$4.00	George T. Rice & Co., Worcester
Curtain rings	2 gross	$0.50	George. T. Rice & Co., Worcester
Britannia lamps	1 pair	$1.33	Henry W. Miller

use of patients, such as fifty bedsteads, purchased at a total cost of $150; 50 "hair mattresses" for $187.50; and 24 "dark common chairs" for $12.

A tour guide of the Worcester State Hospital written in 1983—only a few years after the Kirkbride building ceased to be occupied—described its furniture, which was custom-made by in-house craftsmen (likely including patients), as "very baroque and very interestingly awful" (Tour of the Worcester State Hospital 1983). According to the guide, the common rooms of the hospital were unusually large—particularly the dining rooms, which were equipped to seat 40 people—so that "[s]ome of the furnishings appear smaller than they are." The ordinary middle-class items selected to furnish the first state hospital in 1833 would have likewise appeared out-of-scale with the extended dimensions of the wards, which were intended to house a large "family" of patients rather than the increasingly small and intimate families of the average nuclear family. Such dissonances in scale between rooms and furnishings would have given the hospital an unsettling, Alice-in-Wonderland quality for patients who were accustomed to the modest scale of nineteenth-century domestic interiors.

Yet patients did exercise some agency in shaping their surroundings, as one photograph of a patient room from the early twentieth century suggests. This room is heavily ornamented with wall hangings and ephemera, including small brooms (figure 1.7). The accretion of ornaments imbues the room with a distended temporality, indicating that the patient has been there for some

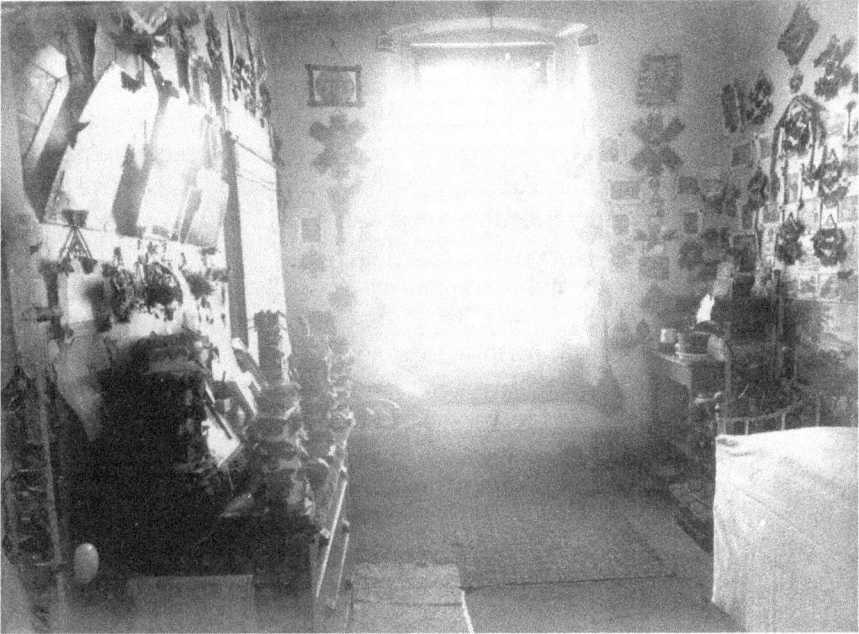

Figure 1.7 Patient Room in the Worcester State Hospital (Early Twentieth Century).
Courtesy of the Worcester Historical Museum.

time, and suggesting a level of permanence and stability in residence that directly contradicts the purpose of the hospital as a curative machine. The ability of this patient to colonize the room, claiming it as a distinctly individualized space within the institutionalized setting of the hospital, suggests that at least for certain patients, the asylum was truly a home in which they could stake out a degree of personalized—rather than institutional—domesticity. For these patients, the material substrate of the hospital could be mobilized to create their own expressions of creativity and memory. Like asylum administrators, they recognized the power of materiality as a medium for communication and a moderator of experience. Yet they contested administrators' monopolistic authority over that power, staking their own claim to control the environment and in doing so, influence their own and others' experiences of the asylum. To these patients, manipulation of the environment was a means of defying institutional discipline that made them the objects, and never the authors, of meaning. Administrators' attempts to control the asylum was matched by patients' ingenuity in manipulating their environments and cultivating their own material worlds within the asylum.

PATIENTS' BELONGINGS

Upon their commitment to the asylum, patients were often divested of many or all of the belongings they brought with them. While purportedly instituted to prevent self-harm, this practice often served to dehumanize patients, undermining their identities and severing ties with the outside world. In his account, Robert Fuller described the trauma of being "literally robbed" upon his arrival at the McLean Asylum. The items that were taken from him— including a "pocket book and notes, money, watch, knife, rule, pencil, [and] hair comb" (Fuller 1833: 15)—were all essential elements of the "identity kit" that enabled patients to perform their social personas and maintain their place in the world. Without these markers of identity, patients were unmoored in an unfamiliar setting, stripped of the tools they used to relate to others and orient themselves socially (Hamlett 2013: 93).

Administrators could mobilize patients' belongings as a means of discipline. Packard reported that when she was on good terms with the superintendent, she was given a large degree of freedom and allowed to keep her "gold watch, spectacles, pocket knife and scissors; books and papers," and could "read, knit, sew, ride, [or] walk" (Packard 1873: 101). Once she started to criticize the administration and pressured for her release, however, she was stripped of these possessions, and forced to mobilize other materials of the asylum for use. She wrote letters and journal entries "on tissue paper, in the margins of newspapers, and on cotton cloth," and embroidered messages into the underwaists she sewed for her daughter (ibid.: 168). These messages were Packard's means of protesting her confinement, and ultimately contributed to securing her release when they were able to reach the outside world.

Other patients took a more direct route of resistance by seeking to remove the physical barriers standing in the way of their liberty. In the *American Journal of Insanity,* psychiatrist J. Edwards Lee itemized the "collection of instruments" that patients at the Wisconsin State Hospital created to facilitate their escapes, including "keys made out of wood, pewter, and wire; files manufactured from old knives; saws from hoop iron; [and] screwdrivers from ten-penny nails. No less skill is shown in concealing their operations, in making fac-similes [*sic*] of screw heads out of bread and covering the different ways the gaps which they have made, until they can get farther opportunity to work" (Lee 1847). Moses Swan recounted that his roommate at McLean, Joel Swain, made a "wooden false key to our room" (Swan 1874: 128–129). Given the meaning with which keys were freighted as symbols of authority, patients' efforts to create their own keys can be read as a means of disrupting institutional hierarchies and contesting the limits of power.

CONCLUSION

Moral treatment was intended to target the humanity within the lunatic, encouraging his or her return to sanity through gentleness and mutual trust with the physician within a holistically therapeutic environment. The strength of this paradigm, and the reason for its widespread acceptance by reformers and the medical field, lay in its persuasive rather than coercive power. While the first asylums, in which the ratio of staff to patients was low, may have come close to meeting this ideal, it quickly became untenable under the circumstances of mass institutionalization and as a result of the particular material practices exercised in the construction and furnishing of the hospital. Asylums were designed as aesthetic objects, which mobilized the cultural currency of Gothic architecture to signal their progressive, modern, and genteel character; yet these qualities were mainly confined to the surface of the institution. In their capacity for physical containment, robust structure, and hierarchical organization, state hospitals such as Worcester more closely resembled prisons than facilities for the sick, revealing their mixed genealogy as both medical facilities and places of confinement. Likewise the Kirkbride plan, while designed as a tool of medical classification and treatment, functioned largely as a means of repression and control, mobilizing the spatial dimensions of the hospital to create an institutional hierarchy that elevated small groups of wealthy patients at the expense of a large underclass of paupers, immigrants, minorities, and "chronically insane." Such arrangements created a lasting material testament to the role of the asylum in creating and upholding social divisions.

The potential of the asylum as a therapeutic institution was thwarted partly by circumstantial factors—such as the restrained budgets imposed by the state legislature, the growth of immigration, and the difficulty of maintaining proper staffing—and partly by the flaws inherent to its design. Massive, monumental, and immovable, the asylum was ultimately doomed to obsolescence by the very qualities that were meant to ensure its perpetual function. The plans made by asylum architects reveal a strikingly myopic perspective that failed to accommodate the possibility for growth and change, reflecting psychiatrists' assumption that the qualities they considered most important to the aesthetic and therapeutic efficacy of the asylum were derived from "natural"—and therefore eternal—principles, rather than the contingencies of contemporary medicine and society. They failed to create effective asylums not because their underlying premise—that the environment was capable of influencing behavior and mental status—was wrong, but because they believed that the criteria for what constituted an ideal environment would never change: that their rendering of the ideal asylum would continue to convey the beliefs in progress and medical humanitarianism with which they were originally invested. Instead, such structures have come to signify a distinctively haunted quality: an aura of hopelessness and decay that has been aestheticized in the modern genre of ruin photography. Such photographs capture the significations that these buildings have come to acquire over time—the accretions of years of abuse and neglect—rather than their original role as symbols of scientific advancement and hope for a cure.

The relegation of patients' graves to marginal areas represented administrators' efforts to stave off such accretions, thus hiding the evidence for the hospital's failures from public view. Yet the steady decrease in the amount of funds dedicated to the maintenance and repair of the hospital building suggests that administrators ultimately capitulated to the atmosphere of defeat that pervaded the institution, an attitude that quickened the rate of the hospital's deterioration. The material form of the hospital and its ideational role as an emblem of moral treatment were locked in a dialectical relationship. The devolution of the former encouraged the devolution of the latter and vice versa, forming a downward spiral of increasing ruin and dilapidation that culminated in the abandonment and ruination of both the asylum and the promise of large-scale institutional psychiatric care.

Patients shared psychiatrists' belief in the agentive and semiotic properties of the environment. However, the effects they reported while subject to the influence of the asylum were contrary to what psychiatrists intended. Acutely aware of the carceral aspects of the asylum, its increasingly poor maintenance, and the stigmatic associations of the imposing building, they complained that the institutional environment functioned more to cause mental disorder than to resolve it. Refusing to accept their own status as lunatics, they viewed the asylum as a site of confinement rather than of cure. Rather than yielding to the ideological and physical forces of the asylum, patients instead made the asylum the subject of their own acts of agency, manipulating its environment to their own ends. As durational and accretional structures, asylums became not only lasting memorials to the failures of moral treatment but also living texts for the inscription of patients' desires and autonomy.

NOTES

1. The Worcester State Hospital's patient population peaked in 1950, when it surpassed 3,000.
2. The declining numbers of private patients suggest that families were less likely to trust their relatives to the Worcester State Hospital as time went on and it became branded with the reputation of a "pauper institution."
3. Notably, even at its inception in 1833, the institution was known as the State Lunatic *Hospital* at Worcester (later changed to the Worcester Insane Hospital and the

Worcester State Hospital). The term "asylum" was purposefully avoided as it implied an institution that was merely a receptacle for hopeless cases. The term "hospital" on the other hand spoke to the identity of the hospital as a medical institution based on the premise of curability.

4. This number represents a small minority of the 2,000 patients who were recorded as dying at the Worcester State Hospital between 1888 and 1907, suggesting either that the majority of patients who died at the hospital during this time were buried elsewhere, or that the records of their burials in the Hope Cemetery are missing.

Chapter 2

"A State of Conscious and Permanent Visibility"

Sight as an Instrument of Cure and Control

The visual design of the nineteenth-century asylum was predicated on two theories. The first was that because the eye served as a "channel to the mind," pleasant sights would elicit positive psychological reactions; conversely, unpleasant sights would elicit negative ones (White 1893: 576). The second was that a given stimulus would necessarily provoke similar psychological reactions between different individuals by virtue of their shared physiological makeup as human beings. Psychiatrists took for granted that the most positive—and therefore therapeutic—sights were those that accorded with their own idealized vision of the preindustrial world. Conversely, pathological sights were those that were removed from nature and thus "artificial": that is, the gas lights, urban streetscapes, and crowded tenements that increasingly dominated the scenes of everyday life (Winslow 1868: 8–9). Because it was believed that the insane possessed particularly keen senses of vision—making them both vulnerable to negative sights and amenable to treatment by means of positive ones (Ray 1863: 323)—psychiatrists emphasized the importance of dissociating the lunatic from the sight of any object, person, or place that held associations with the original circumstances of his or her illness: a dictate that necessitated the removal of the patient from his home (Annual Report 1839: 65). In place of the environments from which patients had been separated, psychiatrists offered the interiors of the asylum as a simulacrum of a domestic sanctuary, composed of the trappings of middle-class life that they thought to be universal signifiers of comfort.

The confidence of psychiatrists in the commensurality of experience as mediated by the senses can be used to understand both the underlying logic of the asylum as it was intended to function and the reason why that logic failed to have its anticipated effect. The variable that psychiatrists failed to anticipate in their design was difference: how the same sights, although perceived through the common human optical system, could produce heterogeneous impressions in different viewers depending on their respective identities, backgrounds, and positionalities within social and institutional hierarchies. The visual environment of the asylum represented a carefully regulated optical illusion, combining an Edenic, preindustrial, "natural" landscape with "home-like" interiors. Psychiatrists expected that the patient's mind would harmonize with these pleasant surroundings, leading to tranquility of both mind and body (Falret 1854: 226). Furthermore, the mechanics with which this transformation occurred were designed to be invisible, leaving patients ignorant of the strategies with which they were being manipulated (Yanni 2007: 9). However, as I argue in this chapter, patients did not embrace the falsified vision of reality that the asylum offered, nor did they lack insight into its moral machinery. In their accounts, patients nurtured their own, alternative visions of the asylum, vested with their own meanings, memories, and beliefs. This is not to say that patients were not affected by their visual engagement with the asylum. On the contrary, they describe many ways in which they were, in fact, deeply moved and transformed by the sights around them—but not in the way that psychiatrists intended. Instead, the realities of confinement, including the loss of freedom and personal autonomy; the stigma associated with the institution and the inescapable presence of other "lunatics"; and the separation from familiar surroundings and loved ones colored patients' experiences more strongly than any other factor. Patients viewed the asylum as a prison from which they were desperate to escape. Its carefully crafted optics not only failed to disguise the oppressive and distinctively institutional features of the asylum but also emphasized these features through the discordance its visual elements struck with patients' feelings of alienation, shame, and homesickness.

The effects of this failure were intensified in the sites where the asylum's aesthetic coherence broke down, and the institution came to more closely resemble the prison that patients claimed it to be. For lower-class patients, those who were confined to its back wards and "strong rooms," and those who came to the hospital in its later decades, when its external facade had begun to crumble and the city had begun to encroach on its environs, the hospital failed to provide even the most superficial impression of rural beauty or domestic comfort. Accordingly, the therapeutic efficacy of the hospital's visual environment was undercut on two levels: first, in the failure of its idyllic image to mold patients' psychological states in the way it was intended; and second, in the failure to maintain that idyllic image consistently across the spatial and temporal contexts that were encompassed in the history of the asylum.

LOCATION

Psychiatrists wrote that a hospital for the insane should be positioned on the landscape in such a way as to maximize the visibility of bucolic views and the exposure to natural light ("Report on the construction of hospitals for the insane . . ." 1851: 79–80). It should be "near enough to high roads, a railway or canal, and a town, to facilitate a supply of stores and visits of friends" but far enough into the country to protect patients from the pathological scenes of urbanization (Conolly 1847: 9). Ascribing curative agency to the environment itself, psychiatrists claimed that "the locality in which the building is erected may be made to contribute to the cure of insanity" (Browne 1837: 182). This confidence in nature as a therapeutic force resonated with contemporary Romantic beliefs that intensified as the agrarian past appeared ever more remote and was enshrined in an aura of nostalgia (Jennings 2016: 192). The same considerations informed the placement of rural cemeteries, public parks, and other landscapes that were intended to mobilize nature as a means of improving spiritual and bodily health.

The paradox of the vision of "nature" conjured by these landscapes is that an elaborate system of spatial and material manipulation was necessary to produce and maintain the appearance of its timeless, untamed, "natural" landscape. In fact, this vision constituted a historically bound ideal that was routed to contemporary literary and artistic currents. The vistas that psychiatrists strove to create could have been borrowed from "a Constable painting or a Wordsworth poem," and were imbued with correspondent beliefs in "rural morality" (Hickman 2009: 438). Though nineteenth-century landscape architects taught that "[n]ature must be humored and aided, not put in a straight [sic] jacket" (Carpenter 1885: 5), this was precisely the effect that asylums would have on both the landscape (figuratively) and its human inhabitants (literally). Through the process of "sanitizing," regimenting, and surveilling nature, the asylum was designed to marshal medicine and morality, vision and behavior, into a singular therapeutic experience (Reiss 2008). However, the efficacy of this experience in treating insanity was dependent on two variables: the validity of psychiatrists' physiological theories linking sensory impressions with psychological states; and the maintenance of the "natural" landscape in perpetuity, essentially stalling the march of time and the advance of modernity.

Both sites of the Worcester State Hospital fit psychiatrists' criteria for the ideal asylum location at the time they were selected, forty years apart. At the time it was built in 1833, the Summer Street property was located on the periphery of the town (not yet city) of Worcester. In 1839, superintendent Dr. Samuel B. Woodward described how the setting of the hospital was calculated to meet every physical and psychological requirement of its inmates:

This Hospital, with its admirable arrangements and accommodations, is a most desirable residence for the insane. Elevated above the scenes of business, and removed from the disturbances of active population, in the midst of a country affording most delightful views and prospects, surrounded by the healthiest atmosphere; the breezes of summer reach us pure and uncontaminated, and the unsurpassed provisions for warmth and ventilation, furnish in winter a temperature as mild as perennial summer; no frosts enter our dwelling, no heat has ever endangered us. We are safe from the inclemencies of winter, the pestilential atmosphere of spring, or the malaria of summer, and in autumn no disease peculiar to the season, has ever molested our family. (Annual Report 1839: 66)

Maps of Worcester in the early 1830s reveal a sparse network of roads, loosely scattered with churches and isolated farmsteads. Man-made structures were so few and far between that solitary trees served as landmarks. A lithograph of the hospital circulated in the 1830s shows a lone carriage passing in front of the hospital, with hills and trees in the background (figure 2.1). An illustration first circulated in the hospital's annual report of 1854—which continued to be featured in reports into the 1860s—shows a similarly idealized vision of the asylum bracketed neatly into a rolling landscape of hills and greenery, with few other buildings in sight (figure 2.2).

However, illustrations positioned at different vantage points suggest the dramatic changes in the hospital's surroundings that were taking place in the

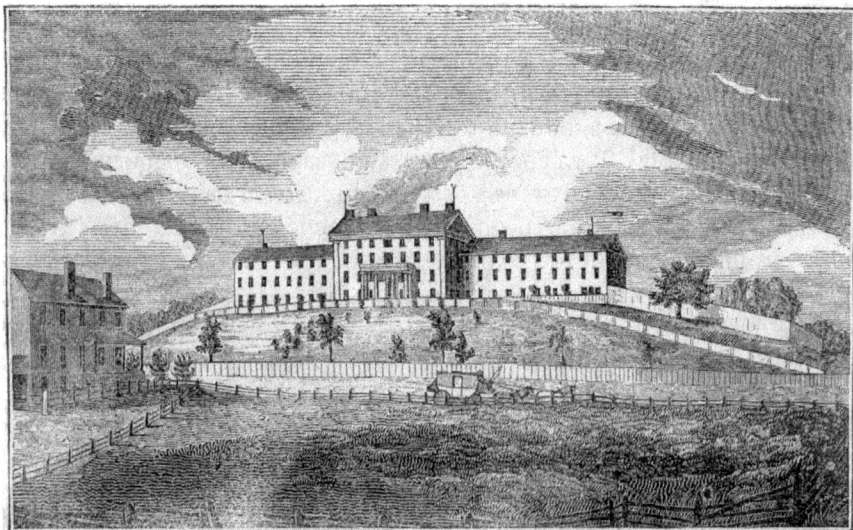

Figure 2.1   The First Worcester State Hospital, Illustrated in the 1830s. Courtesy of the Worcester Historical Museum.

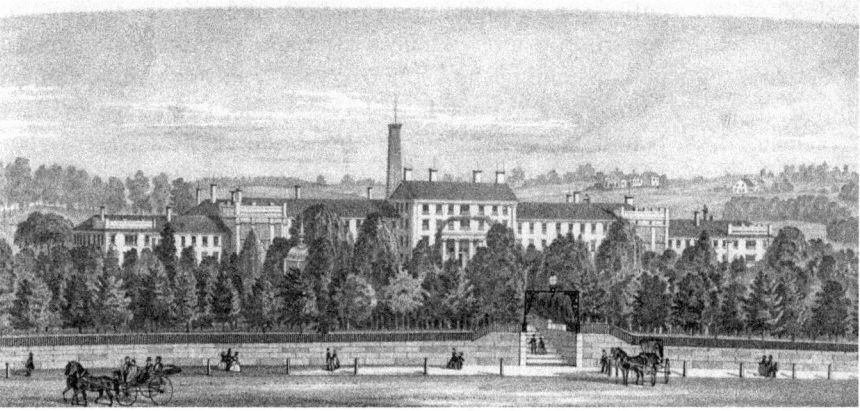

Figure 2.2 **The First Worcester State Hospital, as Illustrated in Its Annual Reports.** A. Prentiss, lithograph, c. 1850–1865. Courtesy of the American Antiquarian Society.

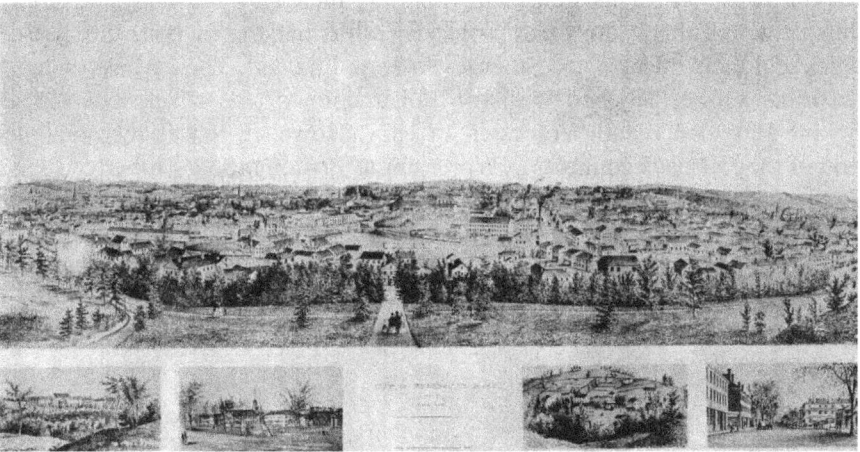

Figure 2.3 **View from the Worcester State Hospital in 1849, Showing the Considerable Growth of the Town since Its Establishment.** The Limits of the Asylum's Property Are Indicated by the Line of Trees in the Foreground. In *Some historic houses of Worcester. Printed for Worcester Bank and Trust Company*, 27. Walton Advertising & Printing Company, Boston, Mass. Courtesy of the Worcester Historical Museum.

1840s and 1850s. A view of Worcester in 1849, looking westward from the hospital's front lawn, shows the considerable growth of the town over the last decade (figure 2.3). The landscape is thicketed with houses and factory buildings, church steeples, and smokestacks leaching plumes of smoke. The dense wall of trees along the hospital's western property line represents a futile attempt to camouflage the encroachment of urban life. Another illustration, published in 1853, shows a train plugging along in the foreground of the hospital, a long trail of smoke marking its wake (figure 2.4). Ironically, the text of the annual reports corroborated these boisterous, congested depictions of the environment surrounding the asylum, rather than the bucolic fantasy shown in their featured illustration. In 1853, less than twenty years since Woodward described the hospital as a quasi-utopian idyll, the trustees wrote:

> The location is such as no one would select for such an object at the present time. The land connected with [the hospital], is altogether too limited, and badly situated; not permitting to the patients that freedom and exercise in the open air, which is desirable in such an institution. The hospital buildings are almost surrounded by city residences, and are not suitable for the uses to which they are put. (Annual Report 1853: 13)

The hospital's founders had failed to anticipate the "rapid growth of the neighborhood" from a "quiet village" to a "busy manufacturing city" (Annual Report 1854: 34). This transformation was fueled by the new transportation networks that connected Worcester with markets in both the coastal cities and their inland intermediaries in New England. The earliest of these networks was established with the construction of the Blackstone Canal, linking Providence and Worcester, in 1827. However, it was the construction of the railroads connecting Worcester to Boston (1832), Albany (1833), and Providence (1848) that elevated Worcester into a major industrial center ("The Blackstone Canal" 2009, Nutt 1919). A stereograph from 1875 shows that the tower of Union Station—built that year, and located only two blocks

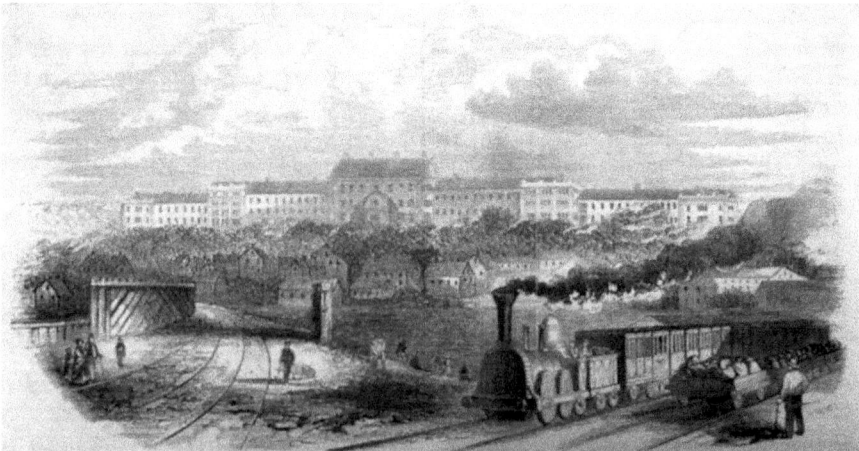

Figure 2.4 View of the Lunatic Asylum, at Worcester, Mass., in 1853, Showing a Marked Departure from the Bucolic Surroundings Depicted in Figures 2.1 and 2.2. Courtesy of the American Antiquarian Society.

away—was plainly visible from the front lawn and southern side of the hospital.

With the opening of its second building in 1877, the hospital was relocated to a site several miles from the center of Worcester, in a rural area that was thought to be beyond the reach of urban sprawl while remaining within convenient distance of the city's amenities (figure 2.5). Photographs corroborate this description, showing wide expanses of agricultural terrain surrounding the hospital, as well as the elaborate gardens and landscaping on its grounds (figure 2.6). Furthermore, the site of the second hospital encompassed a much broader range of elevations than that of the first. While the area surrounding the first hospital was mostly at a uniform elevation, the second hospital was situated at a midway point on a large hill. The effect of this location was twofold. On the one hand, it made the surrounding landscape more visible to the hospital; as a newspaper article announcing the opening of the second hospital stated, the view from the property, "including lakes, woods, meadows, farms, and villages, is admirable, and so far as natural beauty and quiet can minister through the eye to the mind diseased, the unfortunate inmates of this institution will be peculiarly favored" ("An important structure completed"

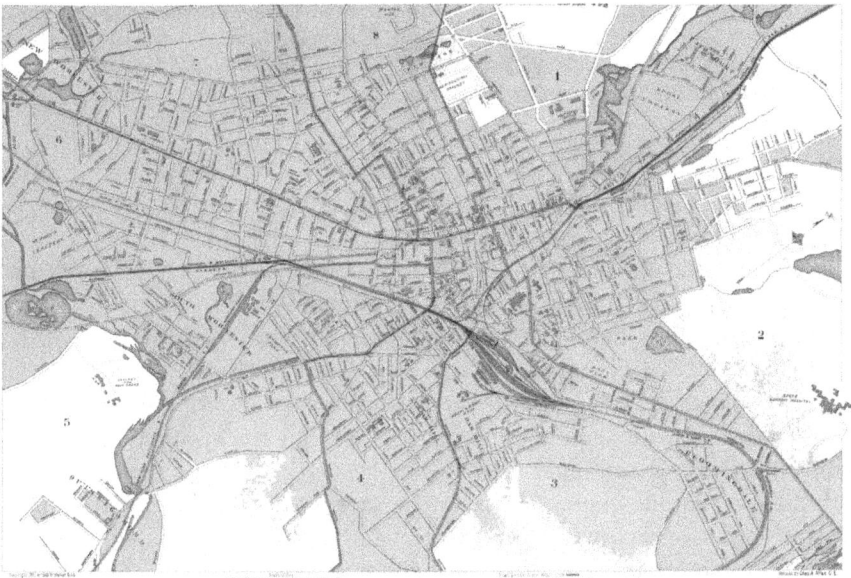

Figure 2.5 Locations of the First (Red Star) and Second (Green Star) Worcester State Hospitals, as Shown on a Map from 1891. By the mid-nineteenth century, the growth of the city had come to surround the first hospital. In contrast, the location of the second hospital was so remote that it is absent from earlier maps of the city (and crosses over the margins of this one). Courtesy of the Worcester Historical Museum.

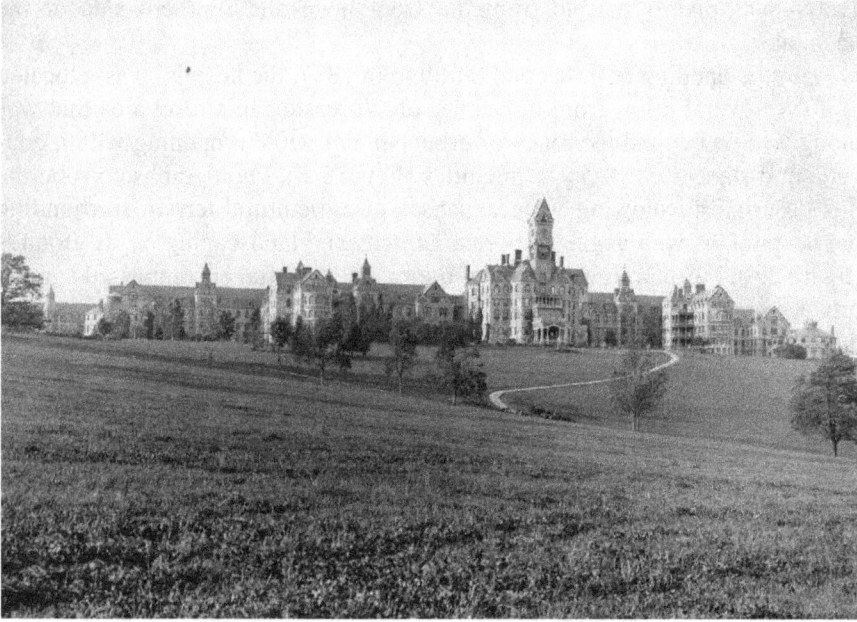

Figure 2.6   The Second Worcester State Hospital circa 1900. Viewshed analysis of the landscape surrounding the Worcester State Hospital projected onto a map of 1870, showing the areas visible from the central Clock Tower (indicated in green). Courtesy of the Worcester Historical Museum.

1877). On the other hand, the relocation also made the hospital more visible to viewers in the surrounding landscape, who could see its sprawling facade and soaring clock tower from miles away.

While the second hospital temporarily remedied the effects of urban encroachment, it failed to anticipate its continuation. This seemingly myopic inability to accommodate change and equip the physical structure for the potentiality of adaptation is a common theme in the history of asylums (Grob 1966). Architects built hospitals for the present, not the future, then scrambled to retrofit their monumental stone and brick structures to new uses and increased demand on an ad hoc basis. Inching the asylum farther and farther from the centers of urbanization represented a futile attempt to "outrun the modern world" (Philo 2007: 114)—the inevitable result of the quixotic mission to resurrect an idealized past as an instrument of modern medicine. By 1908, the administrators of the Worcester State Hospital had come to accept that "the hospital is here to stay, and the city, in its natural growth, must eventually include it" (Annual Report 1908: 12), an acknowledgment that marked a turn in the identity of the asylum and its relationship to the community.

VIEWS

Descriptions of the Worcester State Hospital, and particularly of the second building, which was stationed on a broad eminence commanding a wide vista of southern Worcester, implied that its magnificent views would be enjoyed by all of the hospital's patients. But the prospect from the hospital in fact encompassed an infinite number of different fields of view, inflected by the positionality and subjectivity of the viewer (Dawson 2007). Views would have varied depending on the viewer's location within the building, which spanned 1,100 feet lengthwise. The viewer's location, in turn, depended on his or her positioning within its classificatory system, which combined medical, social, and architectural principles to divine the ideal arrangement of bodies in space. Like many of its contemporaries in the United States, the second hospital was organized along the standards of the Kirkbride plan (Kirkbride 1854). According to this plan, newly admitted, convalescent, and "quiet" patients were housed nearest to the center of the building. Viewshed analysis taken of the site of the Worcester State Hospital, based upon a digital elevation model drawn from LiDAR data, suggests that the central administration building would have commanded extensive visual access to the southern side of the landscape, including the asylum complex and surrounding environment. A viewer situated at the clock tower today can see for miles, into the neighboring town across the lake. The viewer's northern view is more restricted, as the forest provides significant cover. A projection of this viewshed onto a map of the Worcester State Hospital in 1870 indicates that the southern-facing view would have been even more extensive in the absence of modern buildings. The northern outlook, however, would have been similarly restricted, as the forest was in roughly the same configuration then as it is now.

A comparison of the viewshed from the administration building to one taken from the perspective of the Hooper Turret, located at the distal end of one of the receding wings on the women's side of the complex, reveals that the latter encompassed a much more circumscribed visualization of the landscape. While the southern exposure was less extensive than that of the administration building, access to the northern view of the landscape would have been highly restricted. The visibility of the surrounding environment from within the hospital would have been further mediated by the layout of rooms and hallways, the positioning and dressing of windows, and the arrangement of furniture and equipment within the buildings, all of which changed over time with the adaptation of the hospital to meet its changing needs. Lastly, the hospital's views would have become decidedly less bucolic with the growth of the city of Worcester, the erection of auxiliary buildings, and the conversion of meadowlands into agricultural fields to feed the hospital's growing population (Grob 1966). Consequently, individual patient experiences would have been heavily impacted by the spatial and temporal variability in access to what was considered one of the hospital's most valuable therapeutic resources. This variability speaks to one of the central realities of the asylum: for better or for worse, patients' engagement with their surroundings was differentiated by a large number of variables, which produced a corresponding heterogeneity of experiences, complicating and in some cases severely undermining the asylum's function as a curative instrument.

LIGHT

In the nineteenth century, light was weighted with a particular medicinal, spiritual, and semiotic import. It was a "hygienic agent," which exercised a "physiological influence on the development of vital phenomena" (Forbes 1868: vii); it was also a metaphor for reason, spiritual awakening, and intellectual enlightenment. Psychiatrists used the allegorical opposition of darkness and light to articulate the historical transformation in attitudes toward the insane, contrasting the "dark days of error and superstition" against their own "Enlightened views," ever since "brilliant light [has been] thrown on the brain by modern science" (Annual Report 1840: 4). While psychiatrists attributed this change to scientific advancement, the Quaker belief in "Inner Light"—an inherent connection with God that animates every person regardless of mental state—played a large role in reconceptualizing lunatics as human beings worthy of humane treatment (Charland 2007: 67). Even when reason was extinguished, Quaker reformers considered the presence of Inner Light to signal the possibility of redemption; as Pliny Earle —superintendent of the Northampton State Hospital and member of the Society of Friends— wrote in the *American Journal of Insanity*, "in the bosom of the maniac, still burns the beacon-fire that lights him onward towards his home in heaven" (Earle 1845). The result was system of care that retained vestiges of its religious genealogy even as it was increasingly medicalized. When a patient felt a "ray of light . . . penetrate the dark recesses of [his] long benighted intellect," he was experiencing the twinned medical and spiritual effects of moral treatment (Annual Report 1839: 65).

Administrators mobilized the multiple and complementary meanings of light in designing and administering the asylum. Drawing from the treatises of contemporary physiologists, they believed that urban environments shrouded human beings from the vitalizing forces of light, leading to sickness and degeneration, and decried the artificiality of modern life (Forbes 1868: 164). Such statements were haunted by the specter of the rapidly disappearing agrarian ideal. Like the setting of the asylum, light was thought to constitute a therapeutic force in itself, accelerating and sometimes even effecting cures (Forbes 1868: 171; Allmond 2015). The effects of light were not only mental or "spiritual" in nature as Florence Nightingale wrote in *Notes on Nursing,* "light has real and tangible effects upon the human body" (Nightingale 1860: 84). While psychiatrists refuted the long-held notion that the moon itself exerted an influence over the insane (the origin of the word "lunatic"), they suggested that the *light* of the moon was capable of producing physiological effects (Esquirol 1845: 32–33; Rush 1830). Such statements represent psychiatry's continuing efforts to claim territory from the realms of superstition and spirituality, while transplanting many of these earlier beliefs into the biomedical paradigm essentially unchanged.

The hymns used in the chapel of the first Worcester State Hospital, which was completed in 1837 (figure 2.7), further reinforced the correspondence between light as a metaphor for reason and light as a hygienic principle. The lyrics of the hymns held out the hope that light, as both a sensory and spiritual agent, would deliver comfort and even cure those affected by mental illness:

Light and comfort here afford us
Cheer our hearts, our pangs relieve

. . .

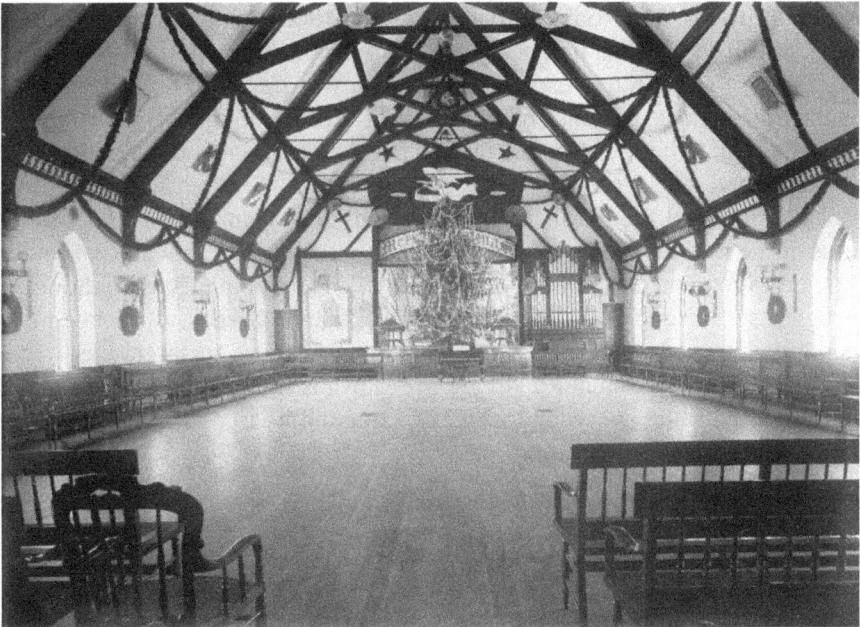

Figure 2.7   The Chapel of the First Worcester State Hospital. Courtesy of the Worcester Historical Museum.

Ascend, O Son of God, thy throne,
Let Reason feel thy sway,
Till in thy light we find our own
And darkness turn to day! (*Hymns* 1837)

While nineteenth-century physiologists wrote that "[n]o amount of artificial, polarized, or reflected light will compensate for the direct sun" (Forbes
1868: 164), some artificial illumination was necessary to facilitate activities
in the asylum after dark. Writing in 1847, Dr. John Conolly recommended
coal gas as the most effective and inexpensive means of lighting an asylum
(Conolly 1847: 37). In some hospitals for the insane, gas lights were kept
low or turned off as early as possible in the evening to save on costs; perhaps
for this reason, the corridors of Boston State Hospital were unilluminated
until 1851 (Frost 1917: 649). Charles Henry Turner, a patient who wrote to
his family from the Taunton Lunatic Hospital in 1877, complained that "I
cannot see to read, after dark; as the Gas Light[s] are too high up" (Turner
1877). The inconvenient positioning of these lights may have been intended
to prevent patients from injuring themselves, such as in the case of a woman
at Worcester State Hospital who "died from self-inflicted burns" from a gas
light in 1894 (Annual Report 1894: 15).

The lighting of the Worcester State Hospital was converted from oil to
gas in the 1850s, and from gas to electricity in 1905 (Annual Report 1850: 5,
1905: 8). Electricity had first been used in an American asylum in 1887, when
the Traverse City State Hospital in Michigan was linked to a plant operated
by the Edison Incandescent Light Company ("Electric light in asylums" 1887:
391). Electric lights were lauded by psychiatrists as an inexpensive, effective,
hygienic, and safe alternative to gas, neutralizing the threats of explosion,
asphyxiation, and fire that had long menaced the asylum. However, descriptions of the new technology in annual reports and professional journals make
little or no reference to any direct *therapeutic* potential in electric lighting, or
in light itself, suggesting—as critics of the asylum charged in the late nineteenth century—that state hospitals had come to function largely as "large
boarding houses" (Annual Report 1903: 13), whose administrators were more
concerned with the everyday logistics of running a large hospital than with
medical treatment or research.

ASYLUM AS HOME

Psychiatrists emphasized the significance of the outward impression that
the hospital imparted to viewers, and particularly to the patient, whose first
impression of the hospital would set the tone for the kind of experience

he or she would have over the next weeks, months, or years. Conolly wrote disparagingly of the "high and gloomy walls, narrow or inaccessible windows, and heavy and immovable tables and benches" that lent early asylums their carceral appearance (Conolly 1847: 7). He urged that a modern asylum should convey an impression "more cheerful than imposing," particularly in its "external aspect," which should "resembl[e] a well-built hospital" (ibid.: 14).

Woodward's conception of the ideal asylum was informed both by his experiences at the Connecticut State Prison and the Hartford Retreat and by his familiarity with asylum literature. In a letter to Dr. Joseph Parish[1] in 1845, he cautioned that a hospital for the insane should not project the image of a prison, but on the contrary, "look as much like a private residence as possible" in order to ease the minds of patients and make them feel at home (Woodward 1845). Furthermore, he wrote, "[c]ourts & high walls give [the asylum] a prison like appearance quite disagreeable to *intelligent inmates*" (ibid., emphasis added). Like many of his contemporaries, Woodward believed that education refined an individual's sensibilities, to the extent that his or her senses were more acutely attuned to the environment. This enhanced sensory capacity could work both for and against educated patients. On the one hand, they were more receptive to therapeutic interventions, as the benefits of positive sensory experiences were enhanced. On the other, they were also more sensitive to negative sensory experiences so that they suffered more by exposure to unpleasant sensations, including the sight of patients who were more insane or less educated than they were. Conolly elaborated:

> If [the asylum] is intended to receive patients of the educated classes, [it] should be situated amidst scenery calculated to give pleasure to such persons when of sane mind . . . Those who faculties have never been cultivated derive little satisfaction from the loveliest aspects of nature . . . When education has called the higher faculties into life, impressions upon them, even from external nature, become powerful for good or ill, and in the case of a mind diseased, may act as remedies, or aggravate the malady. (Conolly 1847: 9)

The annual report of 1857 further justified the differential treatment of inmates on the basis of their families' expectations, starkly positioning the asylum within systems of capitalist consumption:

> Those who pay generously do not place insane relatives here as they find no suitable accommodations; need books, music, pictures, elegant furniture . . . To deprive a man at once of all the refinements and luxuries of good society and reduce him to the cheerless simplicity of a pauper institution would be anything but curative. (Annual Report 1857: 57)

Psychiatrists didn't consider that what made the asylum "homelike" to one patient might differ from another patient on the level of subjective experience. Rather, they considered pleasant furnishings, gardens and recreational areas, and bucolic views to represent features that were necessary to ensure the comfort—and thereby the cure—of patients who were accustomed to a genteel life, but were optional for patients of humbler means, whose personal visions of home were not taken into consideration. These features could include amenities as basic as light. According to Woodward, the halls of the first hospital were "lighted by lanterns suspended from the ceiling, and in those occupied by the *better classes of patients* a large table is placed in the centre of the hall, with lights upon it, that they may assemble around it and pursue their employments, read, write, or engage in amusements or conversation, as they choose" (Annual Report 1839: 89, emphasis added). The need of patients in the "worse" classes for light—whether for recreation, navigation, or the basic ability to perceive the environment—was apparently not considered. Similarly, while the "better" wards of the hospital were "beautified . . . with pictures" (Annual Report 1856: 49), decorated for the holidays, and equipped with pianos, bird cages, and books (Annual Report 1846: 61), the "worse" wards and the basement strong rooms (discussed in detail later in this chapter) were left bare.

Accordingly, when Woodward wrote that the hospital "is a most desirable residence for the insane," he was undoubtedly thinking of the "better" wards and of his own comfortable lodgings in the central administration building, rather than the parts of the hospital that were left unlighted, undecorated, and filthy. The conditions of the "worse" wards were justified by physicians' perception of their inhabitants as uncultured, violent, and insensitive to their surroundings (Annual Report 1837: 14). Such attitudes, and the authority with which they were articulated by psychiatrists, might be seen as evidence of the asylum's function to "guarantee bourgeois morality a universality of fact and permit it to be imposed as a law upon all forms of insanity" (Foucault 1977: 259), as described by Foucault. However, the efficacy of this program of social control hinged on patients' acquiescence, which was hardly guaranteed.

Administrators acted under the pretense that the "homelike" appearances of the hospital would compensate for the reality that the asylum was decidedly *not* home—that in fact, his removal from the most intimate and familiar spaces of a patient's life, and relocation to an entirely alien environment designed to shock the senses back into reality, was deemed necessary for his recovery (Buttolph 1847: 373). The asylum deployed architecture, landscape, and furniture in the fabrication of a vast, immersive deception, rendering the asylum a "home" on the level of its visual surface: a domestic simulacrum. Patient accounts suggest that the asylum most often failed in pulling off this optical sleight-of-hand. Clifford Beers acknowledged that although "[t]he ward to which I was confined was well furnished and as homelike as such a place could be . . . in justice to my own home I must observe the resemblance was not great" (Beers 1913: 47). To Beers and other patients, what made a place a home was not its appearance, but the presence of friends and family, the memories with which material objects and spaces were freighted, and the liberty to behave as one pleased, unencumbered by the stultifying routine and rigid discipline of asylum life. Such personalized and affective conceptions of the home only grew in significance over the course of the nineteenth century, as the domestic sphere was sanctified as a private place of refuge: a true "asylum" for individuals and families (Gardner 1874).

Perhaps partly for this reason—and partly due to the failure of asylums to effect the anticipated percentage of cures—psychiatrists of the late nineteenth century had come to acknowledge the limits of therapeutic architecture in manufacturing a "homelike" experience for patients. In his 1887 annual report, Worcester superintendent John G. Park wrote (emphasis added):

We hear frequently of hospitals being "homelike"—speaking entirely in reference to State hospitals. I confess I never have seen one to which this word in the ordinary acceptation of the term could be truthfully applied. A ward may be cheerful and sunny and comfortable; there may be pictures and carpets and musical instruments; the tables may be covered with books, and the walls painted in pleasing colors; the occupants of this ward may be happy and reasonably contented, *but I have never heard one of them ever say that it reminded him of home.* Thirty to sixty persons do not live in one room during the day-time at home . . . nor are the members of a family constantly changing like the household of a hospital; neither is a home composed of people kept there against their will. (Annual Report 1887: 15–16)

Park proceeded to write that although "pleasant and attractive surroundings" contributed to the number of recoveries among *curable* patients, the number of *incurable* patients, and the impossibility of separating them from the curable undermined this salutary effect. The "wholesome and baneful influence" of the incurable on the curable "is not counteracted by paint or a picture or carpet, or other means of cheer or comfort in the ward itself; it can only cease with the removal of the cause" (Annual Report 1887: 16).

The presence of other insane people was one of the main features that distinguished the asylum from the homes from which patients were removed. Even a person who was diagnosed with insanity could find the sights and sounds of other insane people upsetting; in fact, psychiatrists believed that insanity might make certain individuals—particularly those of the "educated classes"—particularly sensitive to the disturbing behavior and appearances of other patients ("On separate asylums for curables and incurables" 1865: 247). Such unpleasant sights constituted "exquisite torture" to those whose eyes were "rendered painfully sensitive by disease," and could even worsen their illness (Gaston 1877: 12; Skey 1867: 58–59). While acknowledging this fact, psychiatrists maintained that the overall therapeutic influence of the hospital outweighed these negative effects—a conviction that was not shared by Charles Henry Turner. Entreating his family to release him, Turner wrote that "I am disappointed; and do not understand, why I am kept, when Perfectly Well, and in more danger of becoming worse, by remaining; being constantly in Sight of Crazy men" (Turner 1877).

Over time, the "homelike" features of the Worcester State Hospital deteriorated both in theory and in their material manifestation. In the annual report of 1854, the defects of the hospital's living spaces were described by the trustees:

> There are no sunny parlors, no cosy nooks, no cheerful bow windows opening on green lawns; no adornment of the halls, no variety of pleasant sights for the eye, no variety of pleasant sounds for the ear, but, on the contrary—dull monotony in structure of rooms, unbroken by diversity of furniture, [and an] endless extent of whitewashed walls and ceilings. (Annual Report 1854)

Over the next two decades, the asylum's administrators struggled to attenuate the "dark and gloomy" character of the wards under the restrictions imposed by their budget. In 1855, they replaced twenty-four of the strong rooms with "four large, airy, handsome parlors or sitting rooms, finished in plain but neat style, commanding extensive views abroad" (Annual Report 1855: 5). Recesses were built into walls, partitions between rooms removed, and arches added to lighten the halls. The addition of new maps and pictures to the walls was intended to "give the appearance of light and gaiety" and "beguile [patients] of many weary hours" (Annual Report 1856: 49, 1857: 59). The phrasing used in these reports—"give the *appearance* of"; "*beguile* patients"—suggests an implicit acknowledgment of the fact that the asylum was *not* light and gay, and that the experience of confinement was inherently stifling and tedious. Accordingly, in the decades preceding the construction of the second hospital, the changes made to the old building were admittedly superficial interventions, meant to provide a small degree of relief from the monotony of confinement, while leaving the underlying flaws of the hospital's structure unaltered.

ASYLUM AS PRISON

Despite efforts to domesticate the asylum, the voices of patients resound with their perceptions of their surroundings as a prison. Many accounts specifically target the dissonance patients perceived between the interior and exterior of the asylum, and between the asylum as viewed by outsiders and as experienced by patients. They indicate that the *appearance* of the asylum, however pleasant, did not mitigate patients' feelings of imprisonment. As Moses Swan wrote of the Troy Lunatic Asylum in the 1870s, "I have seen gentlemen and ladies visit this main house and walk through the hall adjoining the dining room, and remark how nice it looked, and so it did, but can such a one imagine how he or she would feel locked up in one of those side rooms as I was with a raving maniac?" (Swan 1874: 58). He emphasized not only the disjuncture between different spaces of the asylum but also between the different positionalities of visitor and inmate, and the role of that positionality and its corresponding affect in shaping experience. The despair of confinement inflected his experience far more than the visual appearance of his surroundings. Robert Fuller, recounting his involuntarily commitment to McLean Hospital in 1832, also contrasted the superficial impression conveyed by the asylum against the lived realities of confinement, acknowledging that the asylum had a "pleasant location" and "delightful outward appearance," "but let [the passing stranger] go within its walls: let him hear the groans of the distressed: let him see its inmates shut up with bars and bolts: let him see how deserted they are: how unfit so lonely an abode is for the disconsolate and melancholy" (Fuller 1833: 23).

In *False Imprisonment of Elizabeth R. Hill*, the eponymous author used a multitude of vivid and trenchant expressions to describe the Worcester State Hospital, to which she was forcibly committed in 1877. To Hill, Worcester was a "devilish cavern," a "maniac ark," and a "Stone Ark Lunatic Hell" (Hill 1881: 20). Fiercely defending her sanity, Hill claimed that her commitment was a tactic used by the North Brookfield Railroad to thwart the lawsuit she had brought against them for damage to her property. "Could I speak," she wrote, "my last breath would be that such a crazy ark (which holds so many fearfully lost species of humanity) ought not to have foundation on earth" (ibid.).

That patients might spend years of their lives at the hospital and possibly die there was a fact that patients invested into their perceptions of the building. Swan described the asylum as "a whited sepulchre without," which "within is full of dead men's bones" (Swan 1874: 108), while Lydia Denny likened the experience of confinement to the McLean Asylum—to which she was committed by her abusive husband in 1861—to being "buried alive" (Denny 1862). Elizabeth Packard, another woman committed by her husband, described how she was "entombed . . . .within the massive walls of the Jacksonville Asylum prison"[2] (Packard 1873: 38). During her first months at the hospital, during which she was housed in one of the "better" wards and afforded a variety of privileges, Packard acknowledged that "but for the grated windows, and bolted doors of prison life, I should hardly have known but I was a boarder, whose identity and capacities were recognized, in common with other guests" (ibid.: 102). The pleasant atmosphere and relative liberty did not ameliorate Packard's sense of injustice at her detention and distress in being separated from her family. However, when she began to openly challenge the legitimacy of her and other inmates' commitment as "lunatics," she claims, she was confronted with the dark underbelly of asylum life. Transferred to one of the "worst" wards, she was barred from going outside and subjected to abuse and substandard living conditions. She corroborates Swan and Fuller's sentiments that "a stranger passing through here, knows nothing about the management of the house" (ibid.: 266).

Not all patients were distressed by the sight of the asylum or their confinement. According to his mother, ophthalmologist Jared Willson "was delighted with every thing he saw" at the Connecticut Hospital for the Insane in Middletown, to which he was moved from an institution in Litchfield in 1889, "particularly the building which he thought was magnificent" (Willson 1889). Mary Willson further described the asylum in positive terms, citing the "extensive grounds that are finely cultivated & filled with every sort of entertainment." However, Jared's experience was not representative. To begin with, according to his mother's letters, he was not fully aware of what was going on around him and may not have apprehended his status as a patient in an asylum; since it is his mother who is writing, it is difficult to approximate what he really felt or thought. Furthermore, his upper-middle-class family could afford to place him in an asylum of their choice, in "one of the best wards." Patients who were supported by the state had to contend with whatever accommodation was assigned to them. This denial of choice, more than the furnishings of their surroundings, undoubtedly shaped patients' feelings of confinement.

Mary Willson's attitude toward the asylum suggests that while patients may have viewed the asylum's exterior appearance as an illusion thinly laid over the reality of imprisonment, their families had fully bought into the asylum ideology. Families' investment in the hospital's promise may have been a precondition for committing a relative, as they must have believed—or at least have been willing to convince themselves—that the asylum offered some therapeutic resource or amenity that they could not provide; in the words of Oliver Frost, whose twenty-eight-year-old son Charles died (of alleged mistreatment) shortly after his admission to the Boston Lunatic Hospital in 1865, "I supposed he could be made more comfortable there, than we could make him at home" (Ellis 1866: 59). The ability to select one asylum over another, as the family of Jared Willson did, may have provided additional assurance that they were acting as informed consumers.

The criteria upon which families gauged the therapeutic potential of the asylum was largely consistent with those identified by physicians. Writing to Rockwood Hoar, a trustee of the Worcester State Hospital, in 1905, Ella Tandberg asked for assistance in securing a position in the Soldiers' Home in Washington D.C. for her brother, Hendrick Smith, whose insanity was attributed to his service in the Civil War. Tandberg cited and endorsed the claim of Smith's physician that "with pleasant surroundings . . . he would remain, as he has for several years past, <u>sane</u> to all appearances, but not <u>strong</u> enough <u>mentally</u> to bear any strain." Unable to care for him at home, Tandberg knew that without Hoar's intervention she would have no choice but to commit her brother to the Soldiers' Home in Togus, Maine, which she wrote housed "an exceedingly <u>common</u> class of men—and I know my brother would never be contented to associate with them" (Tandberg 1905). The collaborative efforts of Tandberg, her physician, and Rockwood Hoar in securing Smith's commitment reflect the fact that "the asylum was not the sole creation of doctors or lay reformers . . . but an institution sanctioned by the whole society to meet certain commonly perceived needs" (Tomes 1984: 12). Families' demands and expectations played a much larger role in asylum design and administration than many historians have acknowledged. Patients, however, "did not share in [this] therapeutic consensus," and often viewed their admission to the hospital as evidence of a conspiracy against them, leading to feelings of "abandonment, disloyalty, [and] embitterment" (ibid., Goffman 1961: 133). Defying their physicians and families, they projected their own meanings onto the structures they inhabited. To them, the hospital was a "prison," a "fortress," a "tomb," a "human rat-trap," a "chamber of torture," or as Charles Henry Turner facetiously designated the Taunton Lunatic Hospital in the return address of a letter written in 1877, a "Crazy Hotel" (Bly 1887; Turner 1877).

Patients' conflation of lunatic hospitals with prisons speaks to a tension that runs through the history of the asylum. While acknowledging the shared genealogy of the two institutions, psychiatrists denied that they continued to share defining features and functions. The legitimacy of the asylum as a medical institution and foundation for the discipline of psychiatry rested on the fact that it was *not* a prison. Asylums were curative, not punitive, and their inmates were ill, not criminal (Annual Report 1854: 12, 1862: 30, 1894: 13). For this reason, criminals—even the criminally insane—were excluded from state hospitals in theory (if not in practice), and administrators worked to erase or disguise the stigmata of imprisonment in their asylums. However, they were not always successful. While the "better" wards of the Worcester State Hospital may have *appeared* "homelike" (even if they were not experienced as such), the strong rooms used to accommodate the "furiously insane" in the first hospital were decidedly carceral in nature: "built of stone or brick, precisely like prison cells with grated doors and windows, [and] apertures for putting in food" (Annual Report 1854: 26). Constructed several years after the main hospital, the design of these cells diverged considerably from the stated ideology and design of the asylum. Even when the rest of the hospital was said to be functioning optimally, the trustees wrote that the strong rooms were "unfit abodes for human beings . . . like relics of a comparatively barbarian age" (Annual Report 1854: 26). Cognizant of the transformative agency attributed to the environment, they acknowledged that not only were insane patients unlikely to recover under such conditions, but that "any sane man" would become "furious and violent by being placed therein" (ibid.). This sentiment was echoed by Elizabeth Packard, who attributed her ability to retain her sanity while in the Jacksonville Asylum to her religious belief—"Even a person with a sound mind, and a sound body, could hardly pass through a course here and come out unharmed, without faith" (Packard 1873: 121)—and by Lydia Denny, who wrote after her release, "Physicians express amazement that I did not *become* insane" while committed (Denny 1862). Of the Worcester State Hospital, Elizabeth R. Hill wrote: "Everything in that maniac ark is calculated to destroy a well, noble, pure-minded person" (Hill 1881: 45).

On this point, it seems, patients and psychiatrists agreed: under certain conditions, the asylum was capable of *causing* the very malady it was meant to cure. After all, patients who protested their commitment did not deny the premise that the asylum could manipulate the senses in order to produce certain psychological effects. Rather, they argued that these effects were pathological rather than therapeutic. By the second half of the nineteenth century, psychiatrists had come to accept this argument to some degree. In 1876, Dr. Charles Bucknill acknowledged that "patients naturally come to regard [the prison] somewhat, in the light of a prison" ("Proceedings of the association" 1876: 337). Similarly, speaking at the laying of the cornerstone of the Danville State Hospital in Pennsylvania in 1870, Dr. Isaac Ray stated that "the prison-like aspect [is] inseparable from such structures," and recommended the installation of "objects pleasing to the eye" to mitigate this effect (Ray 1870: 448). In an 1881 issue of the *American Journal of Insanity,* Dr. Orpheus Everts summarized the volley of criticisms surrounding asylums: "American hospital buildings are too large, palatial, expensively constructed; disagreeably monotonous in linear extension, offensively prison-like in aspect" (Everts 1881: 119–120). These statements suggest that it was *psychiatrists* who ultimately came to accept *patients'* visions of the asylum, rather than the other way around—despite the fact that psychiatrists wielded the greatest power to manipulate the material environment of the asylum.

HOSPITAL PALACES AND THE PUBLIC IMAGE

To those on the outside, asylums eventually came to be viewed neither as hospitals nor prisons, but as palaces. Writing in 1837, Dr. W. A. F. Browne stated that the ideal asylum should be "a spacious building resembling the palace of a peer" (Browne 1837: 226). However, by the late nineteenth century, descriptions of asylums as "hospital palaces" and "lunacy cathedrals" were used in a derogatory manner to condemn the profligacy and ostentation of their architects. Ironically, such extravagance did not translate into comfortable accommodations for patients. Rather, "palace hospitals [are] too often prisons, under the form and with the cost of palaces," according to Dr. Samuel Gridley Howe, chairman of the Massachusetts Board of State Charities, who was tasked with investigating the allegations that the Danvers State Hospital was "a labyrinth of folly and extravagance" (Sanborn 1877: 4, 23). Built a year before the second Worcester State Hospital, Danvers cost almost half a million dollars more to construct, despite being "larger" and "built of better materials." A report presented to the Legislative Session of 1876 attributed this wastefulness to the exorbitant salaries commanded by administrators and architects, as well as to the vain striving of the architect to "display his architectural genius" (ibid.).

Discussing the matter at the annual meeting of the Association of Medical Superintendents of American Institutions for the Insane (AMSAII) in 1878, Dr. William Godding admitted that "we have gone within the last decade into the building of too expensive hospitals, stately palaces which do not add to the curability of the insane" ("Proceedings of the association" 1878: 151). While psychiatrists now acknowledged that their hospitals were imperfect instruments at best, they were more divided than ever over the question of what a therapeutic asylum *should* look like. The confidence with which they had invested early asylums with pleasing views and "homelike furnishings" had disappeared, replaced by a fractious debate over how to accommodate the growing number of incurable patients: unfortunate casualties of the asylum's failed promise and a source of perpetual embarrassment to the profession.

Sensitive to the public perception of their hospitals as "objects of suspicion" and "lunatic prisons," psychiatrists were eager to improve the asylum's image, even as they acknowledged the legitimacy of some of the criticisms (Chapin 1883: 38). The "prejudice in the public mind" mattered because it prevented families from committing their insane relatives or delayed commitment until their mental illness had become incurable (Topp 2007: 252). Godding encouraged his fellow physicians to "depart from stereotyped buildings," that is, the long, baroque monoliths that had come to be iconic, and to "make [asylums] more like homes and less like prisons" ("Proceedings of the association" 1889: 260; Godding 1884: 150). To accomplish this dictate, advocates of the "cottage" or segregate system suggested the partitioning of the monolithic asylum into a series of smaller structures, each specialized to a different function and occupied by a small "family" of patients and attendants. For over a decade, superintendent Dr. Merrick Bemis fought to reconfigure Worcester along this system, but his plan was ultimately defeated by the conservatism of the board of trustees, and the second hospital was built according to an architectural arrangement that was quickly approaching obsolescence (Annual Report 1866, 1870).

By the early twentieth century, the asylum had taken on yet another identity: an anachronism. The same visual features that had indexed progress, improvement, and salutary effects to an earlier, more optimistic age had, through the forces of time, the influence of many personal and investigative reports, and shifts in the theory and practice of psychiatry, come to be seen as barbaric and backward. The visions of the asylum produced by patients on the inside had come to subsume the external image projected by outsiders. The decay and ruination of the Worcester State Hospital further contributed to the haunted, sepulchral appearance of what had once been the state's crowning achievement in public health.

WINDOWS TO THE SOUL

In keeping with physiological dictates concerning the healing properties of light, psychiatrists strove to make asylum "galleries light and cheerful," admitting as much natural light as possible (Conolly 1874: 14). Writing in one of the first treatises on asylum design in 1815, Samuel Tuke, founder of the York Retreat in England, lamented that the "cheerfulness of asylums [was] too often sacrificed to security," particularly by windows that were placed "above the level of sight" or made as small as possible to prevent patients from breaking them or absconding (Tuke 1815: 36). The architects of the first Worcester State Hospital acknowledged this dilemma: "[The insane] require light and pure air, but the doors and windows which give light and ventilation to common dwellings, would furnish them with facilities for escape, and with opportunities for inflicting personal injury, or even self-destruction" (The Commissioners 1837: 12). Following Tuke's suggestion, they struck a compromise between appearance and practicality. Like those of the York Retreat, the windows of the first hospital were designed with a double sash: the inner, wooden sash disguising the outer iron one, so as to give the appearance of a "normal" window from the inside (ibid.).

Elizabeth Dorr, visiting the Worcester State Hospital as a tourist in 1841, wrote in her diary that "the buildings looked spacious & airy & the gratings bore so close a resemblance to the usual sashes in windows that as to take away from the unpleasant impression which the narrow cage like grating always gives the effect" (Dorr 1841). Endorsing one of the premises of moral treatment, she postulated that "this simple difference might be beneficial on a morbid mind." Dr. Edward Jarvis, also writing in 1841, noted that the "apartments for the insane" at Worcester measured eight feet by ten and that "in each room is a large window with an entire cast iron sash, the upper half of which is glazed, the lower half is open, and a lower wooden sash, glazed, covers, and precisely corresponds with the open part of the open sash" (Jarvis 1841: 8). The idea behind this design, as articulated by W. A. F. Browne, was to "prevent escape without *appearing* to do so" (emphasis added) (Browne 1837: 187).

Tuke claimed that the carceral design of asylum windows ironically *encouraged* patients to escape due to the feelings of confinement they provoked. In contrast, patients were less likely to break windows that were unblocked and "accessible" because the unmolested view imparted the illusion of liberty (Tuke 1815: 36–38). Patients who were treated like prisoners would act like prisoners. In a similar vein, Jarvis wrote that patients who were treated as trustworthy would prove themselves worthy of that trust, as "the insane, like other people, respond in feeling and manner to the type of treatment they receive" (Jarvis 1872: 20). To Jarvis, who with his wife operated a small asylum in their home in Dorchester, barred windows communicated a lack of trust to patients.

While patients may have felt the weight of confinement regardless of the style of their windows, it is clear from patient accounts that the presence of iron bars separating them from the outside world made the reality of their situation all the more oppressive. Robert Fuller, at the McLean Asylum, wrote of his distress in being confined to a room "where I could see the light of heaven only through iron grates" (Fuller 1833: 13). To another inmate of McLean, Elizabeth Stone, who was persuaded by the superintendent to reside in the asylum under the pretense that it was a boarding house, the iron bars blocking her view of the scenery—along with the "strange appearance" and "peculiar dress" of her fellow "boarders"—were the first clues that alerted her to the deception (Stone 1842).

Notably, the double sash design was not replicated at the second Worcester State Hospital, whose windows featured clearly visible bars, leading Elizabeth R. Hill to describe her journal entries as "written behind lunatic bars and bolts in Worcester, Mass" (Hill 1881: 25). In an undated photograph of a window in the second hospital, every pane has been broken individually from the inside (figure 2.8). The iron grate conspicuously present beyond the glass reveals the futility of this gesture as an attempt at escape. The difference in window design between the first and second hospitals signals a change in

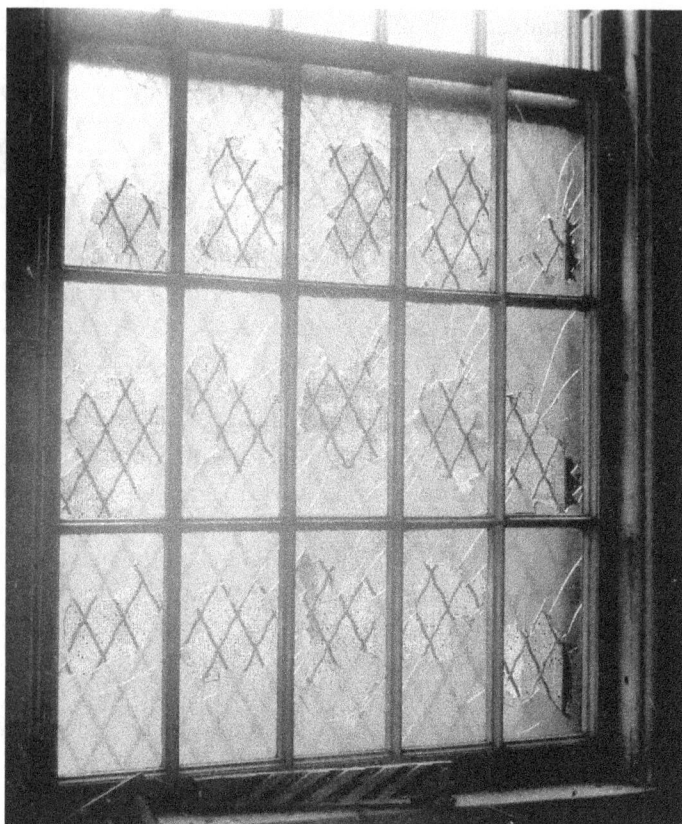

Figure 2.8   Window at the Second Worcester State Hospital Showing Panes Broken by a patient, Undated Photograph. Worcester Historical Museum.

attitude between the early nineteenth century, when patient comfort was privileged above security, and the later nineteenth century, when physicians had begun to accept that their institutions were primarily custodial, and not curative, in nature (Grob 1966: 132; Morrissey et al. 1980: 1–3; Piddock 2007: 223; Scull 1979: 61). However, whether or not their windows were visibly barred, patients had long been aware of the fact that they resided in prisons; the visual trappings of confinement simply served to confirm their conviction.

Nonetheless, the architects of the second hospital were able to dispense with one carceral feature of the earlier building: its high surrounding fence (figure 2.9). Built in the 1850s, the fence had not been intended to prevent patients from escaping, but rather to guard their privacy against the intrusive passersby who had accompanied the encroachment of the city around the hospital grounds (Trustees' Notes 1852). In contrast, the size and remoteness of the second hospital property made a high perimeter fence both unnecessary

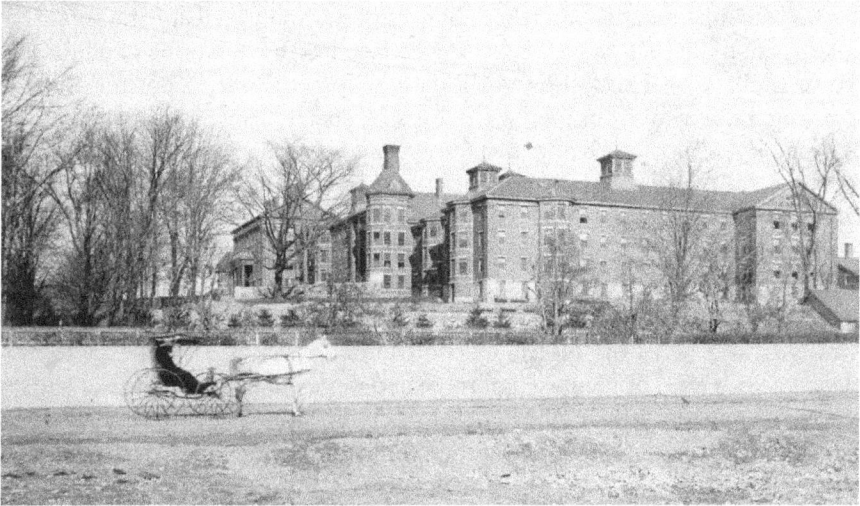

Figure 2.9   View of the First Worcester State Hospital Showing the Surrounding Wall and Fence (Undated; Late Nineteenth Century). The section of the complex on the far left-hand of the photo is the original Neo-Palladian building, constructed in 1833. The section set at a 90 degree angle to the original building represents the extensive additions made to accommodate the growing patient population. Courtesy of the Worcester Historical Museum.

and impractical. Instead, a low stone wall of the kind commonly used to mark agricultural boundaries in New England was constructed using the labor of male patients (Annual Report 1922: 11). The second hospital also featured a long, winding driveway and front gate flanked by granite columns, mimicking the style of a country estate. To avoid giving the impression of confinement, the gate

was never shut (Callaway 2007: 26)—a rather ironic gesture given that windows were barred and doors were locked inside of the building, and that patients who were able to make it to the perimeter of the property could transgress it easily by stepping over the low stone wall. Like many features of the asylum, the rhetorical import of this visual gesture stood at odds with the material realities of confinement.

OUT OF SIGHT, OUT OF MIND

To psychiatrists, the abstraction of a lunatic from her normal milieu and her confinement in an asylum served a multifold purpose. First, it removed her from the pathological sights of her domestic environment and exposed her to new and therapeutically stimulating visual stimuli. Second, it alleviated the insane person's inherent "dread of being exposed and gazed at," during an era when mental illness was viewed as a spectacle worthy of a price of admission (Rush 1830: 236). Third, it provided the family with a safe repository to hide their relative, away from the prying eyes of society. Such concealment was couched in terms of "privacy" for families, who wished to shield themselves from the stigma of insanity. Lunatics were not the only members of society who were hidden in this way: over the course of the nineteenth century, paupers, the elderly, the physically and intellectually disabled, and invalids were increasingly sequestered in specialized institutions that managed, controlled, and effectively erased them from the fabric of everyday life. As John Stuart Mill writes, "one of the effects of civilization . . . is that the spectacle, and even the very idea, of pain, is kept more and more *out of sight* of those classes who enjoy in their fullness the benefits of civilization" (Mill 1836: 130–131). Implicit in Mill's statement is that the relief from the distressing *sight* of others' pain is, in itself, one of those benefits.

Just as the insane were said to fear the intrusive gazes of others, sane people dreaded the gaze of the insane. Historically, the gaze of certain deviant individuals was vested with the power to cause bodily harm. Witches in seventeenth-century Europe and New England were considered capable of "striking down" another person by the "Look or cast of the Eye" (Mather 1692: 255). This supernatural power was transmuted into quasi-materialist terms by psychiatrists who described the physical damage brought about by the psychological distress of seeing "revolting things and sights" (Stolz 1872: 56). Such distressing stimuli were communicated via the senses to the mind, which in turn produced harmful bodily effects. An unborn child could be permanently scarred by its mother's exposure to frightening or disturbing scenes, its physical body imprinted with the stigmata of her mental suffering. In the popular lore surrounding Joseph Merrick, the "Elephant Man," it was said that his affliction was caused by his mother's traumatizing encounter with an elephant during pregnancy (Howell and Ford 1992). Similarly, a mother's "visual exposure" to a lunatic was considered potentially damaging to the fetus (Kromm 2007: 25).

In the 1830s and 1840s, Scottish psychiatrist Alexander Morison commissioned a series of portraits of lunatics for his lectures on the physiognomy of insanity. The 1847 portrait of C. D., a patient at Bethlem Hospital, is rendered by artist Charles Gow using visual allusions to classical depictions of the Medusa (figure 2.10). Her long, serpentine locks, contorted features, and open mouth serve as referents not only to insanity but also to the mythological monster whose gaze holds the capacity to kill. Accordingly, the portrait reifies the conception that "madness was located in the eyes" (Fraser 1998: 45); it also genders this madness in a way that would later be mobilized by second-wave feminists who recast both the Medusa and the hysteric as icons

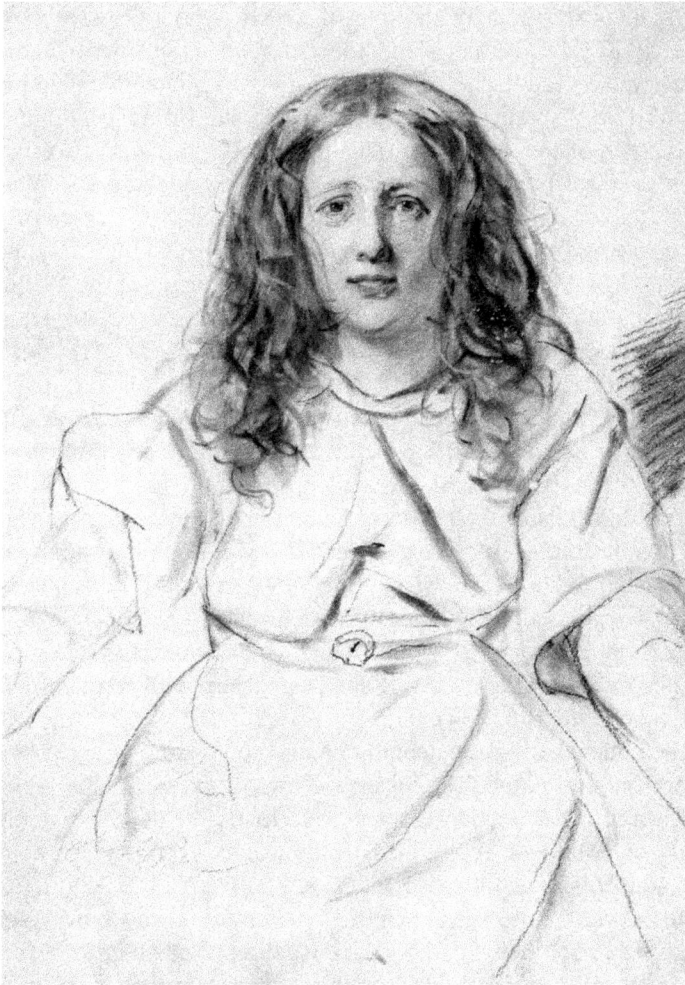

Figure 2.10 Portrait of C. D. Intended to Illustrate Mania, by Artist Charles Gow.
From the Collection of Alexander Morison. Courtesy of the Royal College of Physicians
of Edinburgh.

of female power (Mitchell 2000). The perceived dangerousness of the insane
gaze, whether real or imagined, helped to justify the confinement of lunatics
on a visceral level. In orienting their therapeutics along lines of visibility and
invisibility—mapping the contours of what the insane should see or shouldn't
see, and where the insane should be seen and shouldn't be seen—psychiatrists lent medical legitimacy to this confinement.

Furthermore, early psychiatrists mobilized the seemingly natural repul-
sion of the insane and sane as a means of cure. Benjamin Rush wrote that

"the madman is terrified by the eye of a man who possesses his reason" (Rush 1830: 173). This fear—and the deference it inspired in the insane person—served as the basis for moral treatment as conceptualized by Rush, who believed that "the first object of the physician [in treating the insane] is to catch the eye of the madman." This mechanism of control was said to be have been used by Francis Willis in treating King George III. When asked by a committee of Parliament "what power the Doctor possessed of instantaneously terrifying [the king] into obedience," Willis asserted, "By the EYE!" (Tromans 2010). The "*basiliskan* authority" demonstrated by Willis signals the transformation that Foucault identifies as marking the commencement of "modern" treatment of insanity: "Madness would [no longer] cause fear; it would be afraid" (Foucault 1977: 245). According to Foucault, psychiatrists also weaponized the innate fearsomeness of the insane gaze against itself, as illustrated by Philippe Pinel's experiments with "recognition by mirror." Confronting the patient with his own likeness—in the form of another lunatic displaying similar delusions—forced "madness [to] see itself," as "pure spectacle and absolute subject," an experience that was hoped to shock the patient back into reality (ibid.: 262). Many patients—particularly those who claimed to be sane—expressed their fears of "the insane." On her first night at the Worcester State Hospital, Elizabeth R. Hill was awoken by the night watch entering her room to check on her; she "screeched with terror, for I thought them lunatics" (Hill 1881: 34).

Over the course of the nineteenth century, the power of the psychiatrist's eye to confront and coerce the insane was transmuted into the power of the medical gaze to observe and diagnose. "No longer an organ to ban madness, intimidate, or comfort," the eye of the nineteenth-century physician "only recorded and collected morphological data" (Topp 2007: 296). Later, the diagnostic power of the medical gaze was amplified by new technologies and discoveries, as "new methods of visualizing and recording reinforced the traditional reliance on sight," forcing doctors "to ponder the relationship between sensations and reality" (Bynum and Porter 1993: 2–3). This was a particularly difficult task for psychiatrists, who struggled to identify physiological changes in the brain corresponding with insane behaviors (Leidesdorf 1865; Gray 1874). This failure to visually localize insanity was particularly threatening to the legitimacy of psychiatry at a time when the etiology of disease, through autopsy and microscopy, was being rendered increasingly visible. Physicians could identify the infinitesimally small microbial agents that were responsible for infection, yet they were unable to identify any structural anomaly or lesion to account for paralyzing melancholy or violent fits of mania. Nonetheless, psychiatrists' professional claim to insanity as medical doctors was contingent upon the conviction that insanity was a disease of the brain (Gray 1871).

In the absence of markers in the brain, some psychiatrists attempted to map mental pathologies onto the face, first by illustrated physiognomic studies—such as those created by Etienne Esquirol and Alexander Morison—and later using photography. In 1884, physicians at the Worcester State Hospital created "a large collection of pictures . . . illustrating the positions and features of the different types of insanity" exhibited by their patients (Annual Report 1884). These images served "to construct a readily available visual blueprint from which to abstract mental and social aberrance" (Fraser 1998), rendering insanity visible to the medical gaze, and, consequently, allowing psychiatry to articulate its practice in the accepted medical lexicon of the visual symptom. Because the photographs of patients at Worcester served the additional function as "a means of identification in cases of elopement" (Annual Report 1884: 13), it could be said that the medical gaze doubled as a surveilling gaze, both passively recording and actively controlling the behavior of patients through its omnipresent attention.

The nineteenth-century asylum served the complementary functions of removing insanity from the visual scrutiny of society while simultaneously fixing it within the sight lines of the medical gaze. However, because "patients are never merely subject to or are constituted by the gaze, but interact, respond to, challenge, speak to, and return both the gaze and the glance" (Davies 2007: 312), it is necessary to look beyond the medical field of view to the perspectives of patients who registered their perceptions of themselves and their surroundings. In these accounts, the asylum appears as prison, the lunatic as a sane person. Never "reduced to silence" (Foucault 1977: 250), the patient voice vividly renders its experiences in ways that contest and complicate the utopian illusions of the asylum.

SURVEILLANCE

Surveillance formed one of the major strategies whereby the asylum functioned to "render visible those who are inside it" in order to make them amenable to moral treatment (Topp 2007: 246). Psychiatrists acknowledged that constant observation created a distrustful and oppositional dynamic between the observer and the observed, making the asylum a "complex political space of struggle over surveillance and discipline" (Coleborne and MacKinnon 2003: 21). Browne wrote that surveillance, and the correspondent lack of privacy and sense of distrust, is "painful to the self-respect and sense of honour which many lunatics cherish" (Browne 1837: 149). Nonetheless, it was viewed as necessary to prevent patients from harming themselves, to maintain order, and to instill the kind of self-discipline that would force the insane to adopt new, rational behaviors and habits. When compared with mechanical restraint, considered the only alternative for patients who were uncontrollable, surveillance appeared as the lesser of two evils (Conolly 1847: 27).

Psychiatrists developed a variety of strategies to mitigate the evil effects of surveillance. Conolly suggested that "inspection plates on doors . . . should be noiseless," so as not to alert patients to the fact they were being watched (ibid.). Yet he discouraged the use of "secret openings" for observation of patients in their rooms, stating that patients would be "more offended" by this illicit violation of their privacy "than by more avowed watchfulness" (ibid.). Deception could only be taken so far, not because it was inherently wrong to deceive, but because the "heightened sensibilities" of the insane would alert them to the reality of the situation, spoiling the integrity of the asylum's optical tricks and thereby rendering them ineffective.

At the second Worcester State Hospital, a novel system based on Jeremy Bentham's Panopticon was developed in 1886 to house suicidal patients. Designed by George D. Rand, the same architect who designed the main Kirkbride complex, the Hooper Turret (for women) and the Gage Turret (for men) were two round structures positioned at opposite ends of the hospital's two wings (figure 2.11):

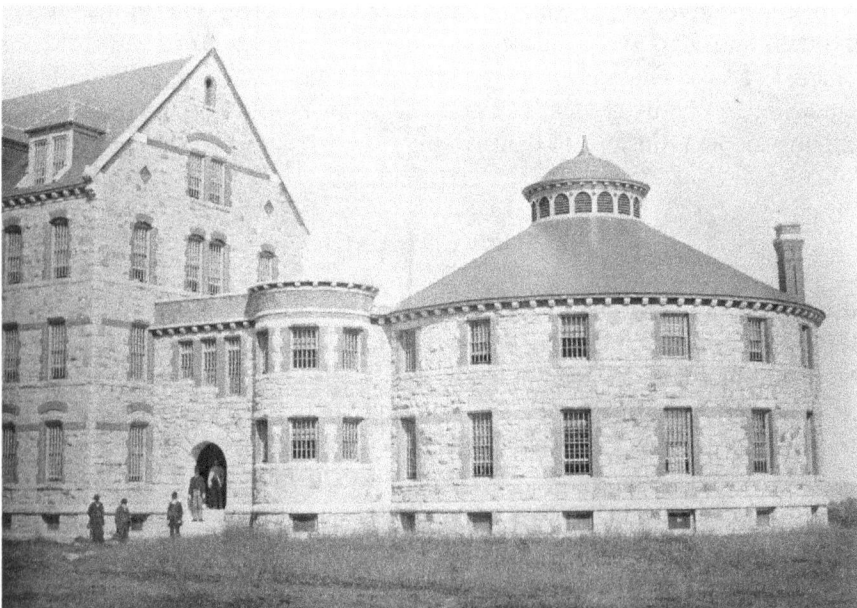

Figure 2.11 The Gage Turret, Undated (Late Nineteenth Century). Courtesy of the Worcester Historical Museum.

Each building is circular, fifty feet in diameter, two stories high and connected with one of the gables of the present structure by a passage-way with stairs upon one side and bath and clothes rooms on the other. It is intended to use the first floor as a day-room and the second floor as a dormitory. By this arrangement twenty-four persons will be accommodated in each building. By making some changes in the adjoining ward of the present building, a special dining-room is obtained. (Annual Report 1886: 18)

These wards are of novel design, and we believe them admirably suited to their purpose. The patients occupying them are under the constant and uninterrupted observation of the attendants. The cheerful and beautiful room in each ward in which the day is spent must contribute materially to the welfare of this most unfortunate class of our inmates. (Annual Report 1887: 6)

The interiors of the Turrets were said to be "light, airy, painted in harmonious colors, and as cheerful as the nature of the malady of the persons who occupy them will admit" (Annual Report 1887: 15).

Despite the centrality of the Panopticon to historical understandings of strategies of social control within nineteenth-century institutions, there were few actual Panopticons constructed, and even fewer in hospitals. For the most part, the radial system, used in certain hospitals and prisons in the United Kingdom and United States, came the closest to approximating a Panopticon-style architectural system (Skålevåg 2002: 52–53). At the time the Hooper and Gage Turrets were built, the trustees of the Worcester State Hospital knew of only "one or two other similar institutions" that had circular wards, including the newly built general hospital at Antwerp, and few seem to have been built since (Annual Report 1887: 15). Notably, one of these rare examples was located in Worcester, less than a mile away from the Worcester State Hospital, along the same street. The circular building was built in 1892 as an addition to the Worcester Memorial Hospital (Annual Report of the Memorial Hospital 1922). Like the Hooper and Gage Turrets, the Memorial Panopticon had two stories, each featuring an open floor plan: the first story serving as a ward for women, and the second story as a ward for children (ibid.).

The design of the Turrets was intended to render the activities of patients visible to their attendants and thereby reduce the risk of bodily harm. However, this design also rendered patients more visible to each other. Most of the accommodations in the second hospital were single rooms, wherein patients could stake out some degree of privacy. In the Turrets, however, patients were more exposed to each other, making them vulnerable to the kinds of contaminating influences identified by John G. Park and by Charles Henry Turner, who believed his mental state was endangered by the "Sight of Crazy Men." Like their counterparts today, nineteenth-century psychiatrists recognized that suicidal impulses can be contagious (Sweetser 1850: 290;

Palmer 1878: 448); Isaac Ray wrote that even written "accounts of suicide [can] spark imitations" (Ray 1863: 239). For this reason, Dr. Henri Falret warned that "bringing together the suicidal might be fatal by contagion of example" (Falret 1854). Either the administrators of the hospital did not recognize this possibility, or they believed that the risks of this arrangement outweighed the potential benefits. Faced with a perpetual staff shortage, it made logistical sense to congregate a large number of suicidal patients under the watchful gaze of a few attendants, rather than allocating a single attendant to watch over each suicidal patient in his or her individual cell. It was also expected to relieve some of the necessity of restraint, a practice that was increasingly disparaged inside and outside of psychiatry (Annual Report 1840: 80). While these reasons were often used to justify the use of dormitory-style wards for suicidal patients in asylums, the Worcester State Hospital was the only institution in which a Panopticon-style building was used to amplify the effects of surveillance.

   While enabling more effective observation, the unique design of the Turrets made them less homelike in structure than the other parts of the hospital. Their open spaces were larger than the rooms of the typical nineteenth-century house, and their distinctive shape provided an inescapable reminder of their function as instruments of surveillance. Furthermore, the dormitory-style layout provided little opportunity for patients to personalize their own spaces within the hospital, as was possible for those who occupied single rooms (see chapter 1). Nonetheless, administrators made concerted efforts to domesticate the Panopticon. One photo, featured in the 1888 annual report, shows the interior of the first story of the Hooper Turret, which served as a day room for suicidal women. The walls are hung with photographs and fitted with contrasting wainscoting; rocking chairs and small tables with patterned tablecloths are spread throughout the room; and the central platform, buttressed by Corinthian columns, features a potted plant and old-fashioned spinning wheel. A second, undated photograph shows the sleeping quarters of one of the Turrets decorated for Christmas, the central column of the platform looped with greenery, and festive garlands overhanging the circle of neatly made beds (figure 2.12).

CONCLUSION: OPTICAL TRICKS
AND MYOPIC VISIONS

While psychiatrists discouraged outright dishonesty, stating that "deception [was] destructive to the welfare of patients" (Annual Report 1867: 65), the very basis of moral treatment was founded on deceit, or more accurately, an elaborate illusion. Drawing from early modern conceptions that regarded the

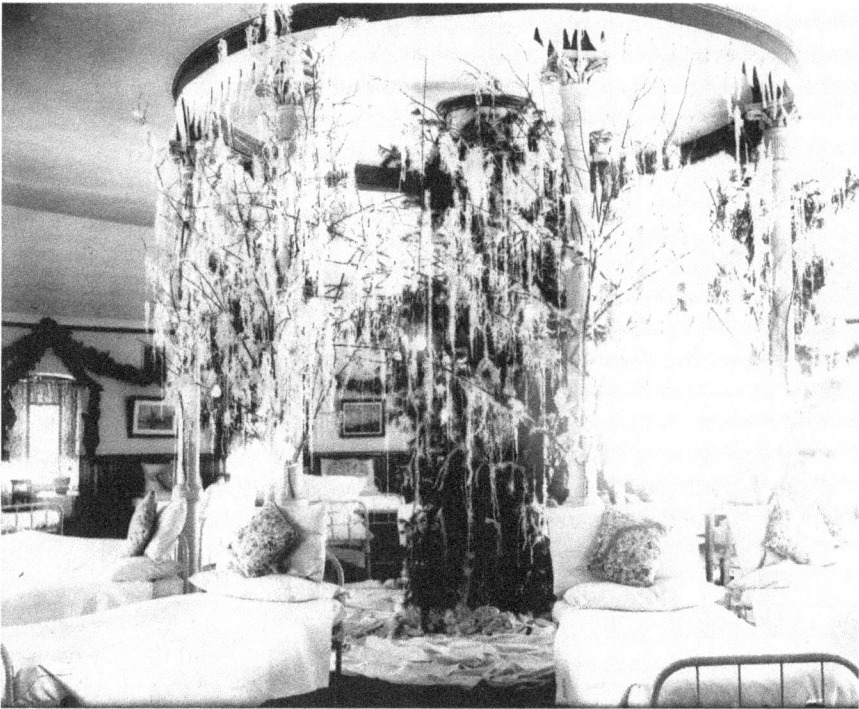

Figure 2.12   Interior of the Hooper Turret Decorated for Christmas. Courtesy of the Worcester Historical Museum.

eye as the "channel to the mind," psychiatrists believed that lunatics' behavior could be shaped by their engagement with the visual world. Accordingly, the fabrication of the asylum as a series of "homelike" interiors, lodged in an idealized natural landscape lifted directly from Romantic art and literature, would "beguile" the patient into a state of mental harmony, essentially tricking him or her into wellness.

The efficacy of this illusion was undermined by several factors. To begin with, psychiatrists' visions of both "Nature" and "Home" were specific, not universal, tied to historical and class-based contingencies; accordingly, they were targeted at a certain kind of patient, the "educated" lunatic who would receive certain kind of treatment. Other patients—the "furious," "violent," and uncultured—were relegated to spaces that administrators acknowledged were "prison-like" and fundamentally unfit for human habitation. The hospital's therapeutic resources were thus unequally distributed, with a vast chasm separating the "best" from the "worst" accommodations. However, even those patients who occupied the "best" wards failed to accept the mirage conjured by the asylum. Their accounts register their distress at their confinement and the consistent perception of their surroundings as a prison. While they agreed with psychiatrists that the environment could shape mental health, they maintained that the environmental forces at work in the asylum were pathological rather than therapeutic. Similarly, while patients shared psychiatrists' conception of the home as a salutary and sanctified place, they disagreed as to what constituted a home. Pleasant furnishings and views, books and pianos, and maps and pictures failed to convince patients that they were anywhere but an institution, particularly when they were confronted by the sights and sounds of other lunatics. Accordingly, patients' affective states largely shaped their visual perception of the asylum, rather than the other way around.

Patients' failure to accept the optical trickery of the asylum undermines Foucault's thesis that the asylum operated as a mechanism of social control. While the control and containment of deviancy may have been the objective of the asylum, its success was thwarted by the fragility of its visual conceits when placed under the scrutinizing gaze of the distressed and indignant patient. Such individuals were quick to identify the disjunctures between the appearances of the asylum, particularly to outsiders, and the reality of their lived experiences within its walls. Over the years, as the asylum's image deteriorated through the physical decay of the buildings and the inescapable presence of the "incurable" insane, psychiatrists' attitudes came to echo those of their patients. By the late nineteenth century, even they had to admit that the asylums they had imagined were only an illusion, thinly spackled over an increasingly untenable reality. As Browne wrote, "a perfect asylum may appear to be a Utopia; 'a sight to dream of, not to see'" (Browne 1837: 176).

NOTES

1. Parish was a physician in Burlington, New Jersey, who would go on to found the American Association for the Cure of Inebriety and the *American Psychological Journal*.

2. Both Denny and Packard were ultimately declared sane by the courts and released.

Chapter 3

"As Syllable from Sound"
The Sonic Dimensions of Confinement

Just like sights, pleasant and unpleasant sounds were vested with the capacity to respectively help or hinder the recovery of patients in the asylum. The ear, like the eye, was believed to be routed to the mind. According to the nineteenth-century German physiologist Hermann von Helmholtz, hearing was "nothing less than a bodily form of sympathetic vibration, and the ear a kind of microscopic Aeolian harp wired to the brain" (Picker 2003: 87). When the ear vibrated in tandem with comforting music or the relaxing sounds of nature, it imparted harmony to the mind. On the other hand, when the strings of the Aeolian harp were seized by the dreadful cacophony of urban noise or other distressing noises, psychological torment was sure to follow.

Psychiatrists believed that insanity could be triggered by exposure to discomfiting sounds. Loud, strident noises of any kind were thought to incite irritation in the brain, which could distort perception and sensation, "commit great ravages in the region of the intellect, and bring about a considerable impairment of its integrity" (Griesinger 1866: 318). The "constant noise" of urban environments and industrial production, "which shakes the nervous system, disturbs the sleep, [and] engenders the habit of nervous irritability," was believed to be particularly damaging to both mental and bodily health (Taylor 1871: 64–65). Yet pathological sounds could also be found far outside the city. In the second half of the nineteenth century, settlers of the Great Plains were said to suffer from "prairie madness," a type of insanity that was attributed to their exposure to the incessant sound of "wind running on the plain" (Velez 2018). Even endogenous noises—such as incessant ringing or buzzing in the ears caused by "aural disease"—could provoke such distress in an otherwise healthy person that he or she might contemplate suicide ("Mental afflictions and aural disease" 1888: 410).

Insanity was thought to render individuals particularly sensitive to sound. For this reason, superintendent Dr. Samuel B. Woodward wrote that "during period[s] of high excitement, the mind should be kept quiet, secluded from company and noise" (Annual Report 1835). A placid environment allowed the "mind [to be] more easily controlled, as new impressions from the outward world are excluded" (Stolz 1872: 107). "Absolute rest and quiet" served the purpose of "placing the brain in splints," as though it were a broken limb that needed to be held straight until it healed. The mind would be held in such an arrangement until it was permanently molded to that form (White 1893: 571). For this reason, the asylum was designed to shut out the noises of the rest of the world, particularly those that arose from the insalubrious scenes of industrialization. At the same time, the asylum was designed to function as an echo chamber in which the gentle, instructive sounds of moral treatment would reverberate, stimulating patients to adopt new, healthy thoughts and behavior. The ear, a "proficient moral educator," was equipped to absorb the lessons imparted by the institution (Stolz 1872: 80).

As an "acoustically resonant space," consisting of "plastered walls, stone and brickwork combined with stone or wooden floors," the asylum as a material entity was designed to aid in alternately eliminating and amplifying sound in order to exert particular effects on the body and mind (MacKinnon 2003: 75). The soundscape of the asylum thus represented "simultaneously a physical environment and a way of perceiving that environment . . . both a world and a culture constructed to make sense of that world" (Helmreich 2007: 623; Thompson 2002: 1; Feld and Brenneis 2004). However, the distinctive patterns of silence and noise that resulted did not always conform to psychiatrists' designs. Because "the aural was a fundamental site of power contestation," psychiatrists and patients were constantly engaged in competing tactics for the control of the asylum soundscape (Brian 2012: 307). While psychiatrists' strategies were targeted at rendering the patient population "quiet"—and therefore orderly and controllable—patients fought to keep their voices and minds from being lost in the din.

"A QUIET HAVEN"

Psychiatrists' intention to construct the asylum as a "quiet haven," set apart from modern life, marked them as "the inheritors of the Romantics' preoccupation with the sublime force of music and quiet of nature" (Cherry 1989; Tuke 1815). In contrast with the salubrious sounds of rural environments, the noises of urban streets "came to be represented as threatening pollutants with noxious effects" (Picker 2003: 66). Psychiatrists nostalgically compared these conditions to the "quiet homespun life of our forefathers" in the "rural districts of New England" ("Restraint in British and American insane asylums" 1878: 531). These forefathers, it was believed, did not suffer from mental illness at the same rate or severity as people of the nineteenth century, living under the tumultuous conditions of modern civilization.

Yet the asylum at Worcester was soon confronted with the very effects of urbanization that it was designed to escape. As early as 1838, administrators complained about the noise that accompanied the growth of Worcester, attributing the "turbulence" of patients' behavior to "the exposed situation of the hospital to the noise of a busy and populous city" (Annual Report 1873: 2, 1868: 3). They lamented the bustle of nearby markets and the intrusion of passersby that "deprived [the] location of quiet," and even resented the "noisy demonstrations of Independence" that "molested" the sleep of their patients every Fourth of July (Annual Report 1870: 8). Such complaints distinguished these men as members of an elite class that increasingly sought refuge from the tumult of urban spaces, either by maintaining country estates outside of the city, or in the case of the Scottish writer Thomas Carlyle, by attempting to carve out a bastion of quiet within the city itself. Carlyle dedicated months and large sums of money in an attempt to soundproof the study in his house in London's upscale Chelsea neighborhood. With "double walls [and a] slated roof with muffling air chambers beneath," this room represented "a professional seizure of urban space, an architectural tactic by which to expel the threat of the noisy rabble" (Picker 2003: 43). It also represented a kind of asylum in microcosm: a "quiet haven" set apart from the city, which was intended to provide the inhabitant's mind a welcome respite from offensive noises.

Like Carlyle, the administrators of the Worcester State Hospital found it difficult to stifle the commotion of urban noise around them and ultimately decided to relocate the asylum altogether. The opening of the second hospital in 1877, "entirely away from the distracting noises and unhealthful smoke and exhalations of the city," was expected to elicit a dramatic improvement in the mood and behavior of patients ("An important public structure completed" 1877). The location—described as an "easily accessible, quiet neighborhood occupied by respectable agriculturists, [with] beautiful scenery in every direction" (Annual Report 1869: 6)—held out the promise of the healing powers of the mythologized agrarian past. To further fortify the hospital's interiors against noise both outside and inside the asylum, the walls were made "of brick, solid and of unusual thickness" (ibid.). The reprieve from the noise of urbanization lasted only a few decades, after which the growth of Worcester caught up with the hospital once again.

SOUND AS CLASSIFICATORY MECHANISM

More than any type of exogenous noise, psychiatrists were concerned with the sounds produced by patients themselves (Ray 1846: 372–374). Under the organization of the Kirkbride plan, the second Worcester State Hospital was designed to organize and manage the different intensities of noise within its walls. The relative intensity of sounds produced by the patients was used as a primary criterion by which they were organized within the hospital space: the quietest near the center, closest to the administration building, and the loudest at the distal ends, with sequential gradations between. This differentiation would have heavily impacted patients' individual experiences of sound within the asylum, leading to the creation a multiplicity of soundscapes, each imbued with its own particular characteristics and associations.

Classification of patients was considered essential to creating and maintaining a therapeutic environment. Exposure to "noisy, excitable, foul-mouthed maniac[s]" was considered potentially damaging to quiet, sensitive patients. Likewise, exposure to incurable patients could hinder the recovery of patients suffering under temporary derangement: "[a] case of acute mania should not be kept awake at night by the noise of a patient suffering from chronic mental disease" ("Proceedings of the association" 1890: 210). To psychiatrists, quiet and docile patients appeared more receptive to treatment; accordingly, such patients were placed in the best wards and singled out for individualized attention in order to give them the best chance of recovery. Noisy patients and those who resisted being controlled were more likely to be seen as incurably insane and to be relegated to the areas of the hospital—such as Worcester's strong rooms—where few or no therapeutic interventions were practiced.

The "incurable but quiet" patient represented a hybrid between these two extremes. While these patients might never be sane, they could be the next best thing: "useful" (Stearns 1884: 27–28). Accordingly, patients who were considered "chronically insane" but were able to perform some kind of labor were assigned a different role in the asylum hierarchy than those who were incurable, noisy, and unable to work. At the Willard Asylum for the Chronic Insane in New York—established in 1869 as the country's first dedicated institution for the incurably mentally ill—patients were divided into two major classes: the "quiet, cleanly, and industrial" and the "excited, paroxysmal, [and] grossly demented" (Dwyer 1987: 132). The latter were shuttered into secure rooms in the main asylum building, while the former were allowed a relative degree of liberty, housed in small dwellings on the hospital property, and charged with various domestic and agricultural tasks. While few of Willard's "incurable but quiet" patients would ever leave the asylum, their relative tranquility made them ideal subjects for the institution's carefully controlled, routinized system of labor, reassuring psychiatrists that even an institution that was not curative could offer some sort of utility ("On separate asylums for curables and incurables" 1865).

NOISE CONTROL AND SEPARATION

While the noisiness of an individual patient was seen as an index of his or her mental state, the patients' collective noisiness was seen as an index of the efficacy of the hospital itself as a curative—or at least pacifying—instrument. Quiet was attributed to effective management and spatial organization, while noisiness indicated some flaw in the system, which psychiatrists most commonly attributed to the size of the patient population and the need for additional buildings to accommodate them. This view was shared by the trustees, whose accounts of the Worcester State Hospital taken during their monthly visits most commonly concerned whether the asylum was "quiet" or "noisy." As William Lincoln wrote in the trustees' notes of December 1838, "[t]he hospital was remarkably quiet, and except for two or three cases of excitement, the institution had little resemblance to the character of an insane asylum" (Trustees' Notes 1838, emphasis original). A well-functioning asylum was one in which the distinctive sounds of insanity were dampened; an ideal asylum did not look or sound like an asylum at all.

American psychiatrists visiting European asylums were amazed by the "extraordinary quiet" they found there, contrasted with the "uneasiness and agitation" of their home institutions (Godding 1877: 542). Some attributed this difference to the existence of a distinctively American or "New England type of insanity," "characterized by intensity," "delight[ing] in noise—the crash of glass is music in its ears" (ibid.). The character of this "type" of insanity was said to be inflected by the inherently freedom-loving "spirit of the American patient," who "madly beat[s] against the bars of his prison-house." In contrast, American psychiatrists envisioned that the quiet English asylums were populated by emaciated peasant laborers who were "relieved from unremitting toil." Yet they also acknowledged that much of the noise of American madness was attributable to the "irritable mental states of patients who have real or fancied grievances against the powers who control or restrain them" ("The favorable modification . . . " 1895: 454). "A visitor in passing through one of our asylums," wrote Isaac Ray in the *American Journal of Insanity,* "is besieged by persons who fill his ears with the bitterest complaints, representing themselves as the victims of the grossest injustice, and importuning him to procure their discharge" (Ray 1846: 342). The legitimacy of these complaints and requests was largely disregarded by psychiatrists who chose to see them only as evidence of insanity. Psychiatrists' proposed solution—that they work to nurture "a better feeling between patient and institution"—was targeted primarily at the maintenance of "quiet and order" and not at legitimizing and addressing patients' needs for their own sake ("The favorable modification . . . " 1895: 454).

While the ideal asylum was a "regulated and regimented soundscape," overcrowding compromised the sonic classification of patients, leading to the indiscriminate mixing of "noisy" and "quiet" (MacKinnon 2003: 75). This mixing was a concern for the Worcester State Hospital's administrators from the beginning. In the first annual report, Woodward wrote that "a separate dwelling for convalescents, and a quiet and orderly class of patients, is extremely desirable. They would then avoid all those disagreeable scenes, and be out of the noise and confusion which they now witness, and from which they constantly suffer" (Annual Report 1833: 8). The disruption of the "quietude" needed by certain patients was thought to constitute a "positive injury" to their bodily and mental health (Annual Report 1845: 6). Ultimately, administrators dealt with this problem not by cloistering the quiet, but by segregating the noisy. The construction of the hospital's strong rooms in the late 1830s (figure 3.1) was intended to "promote the comfort of the more quietly disposed patients by removing from their wards those more excited" (Annual Report 1848: 5). Psychiatrists were not the only ones who objected to the

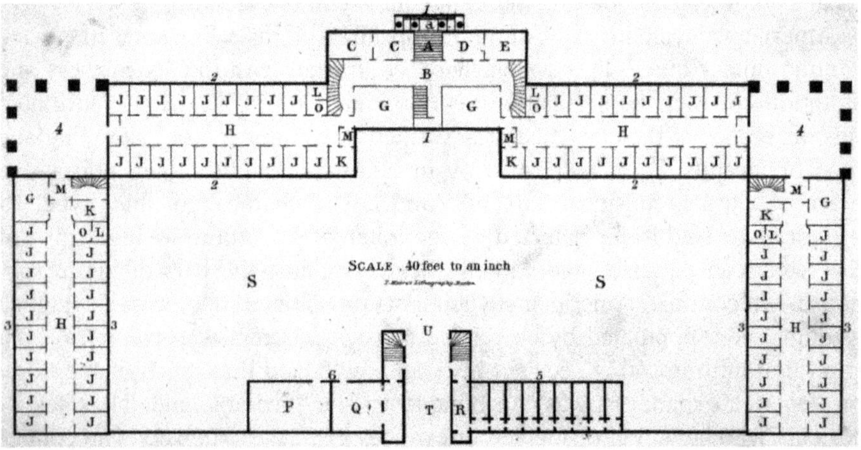

Figure 3.1   Plan of the Principal Story of the State Lunatic Hospital, Circa 1836. The solitaries or "strong rooms" (5) were intended to isolate the noise of the asylum's most "excited" patients from the relatively quiet patients in the main complex. T. Moore's Lithography, Boston. Key: 1. Centre building. 2. Frost Wings. 3. Lateral wings. 4. Porticoes. 5. Solitaries. 6. Wash and store rooms. A. Entrance. B. Hall. C. Parlors. D. Office. E. Dining room. G. Patients' dining rooms. H. Halls. J. Room for patients. K. Attendants' rooms. L. Sink and bathrooms. M. Passages. O. Water closets. P. Wash room. Q. Store room. R. Passage to solitaries. S. Enclosed area, 2200 square feet. T. Arched passage way. U. Proposed chapel. *Source:* Courtesy of the American Antiquarian Society.

mixing of noisy and quiet patients. Describing conditions at the Troy Lunatic Asylum, Moses Swan wrote that his ward was populated by

> a mixed multitude of many nations, of high and low degree, of different faith and different belief, some mild and gentle, whilst others were lion-like and ferocious as tigers; here the quiet ones had to share the abuses of the ruffians, and the ruffians had to share the abuses of the attendants. (Swan 1874: 53–54)

Writing in 1815, Samuel Tuke cautioned that although it was necessary to isolate certain patients who were "extremely noisy and violent" in soundproofed rooms, these accommodations should not be placed in a separate building, as attendants would be more likely to neglect and abuse patients when removed from the regular observation of physicians and the superintendent, writing that "[t]he evil of noise is not so great as those of filth, starvation, and cruelty" (Tuke 1815: 19). Nonetheless, for the sake of noise control, many administrators did segregate noisy patients into buildings far from the main asylum, leading to the consequences that Tuke envisaged. The spatial segregation of the strong rooms at Worcester enabled the trustees to compartmentalize them from the rest of the asylum. Notes from their visits to the hospital from the mid-nineteenth century regularly report that "[a]ll the halls and apartments were found to be in usual good order, thoroughly clean and well ventilated," *except* for the strong rooms, which were "offensive," "noxious," "disgusting," and generally unfit for human habitation (Trustees' Notes).

While it was considered "unfair to disturb the comfort and welfare of quiet and orderly [patients] by thrusting upon them the excitable and disorderly," the influence of noisy patients on each other was either ignored or justified. Dr. George Parkman believed that "[p]lacing boisterous patients within hearing of each other is often useful," as "fear of each other calms extravagant excitement," to the point that they "beg to be removed from such frightful noise" (Parkman 1817: 17). In this way, Parkman envisioned the practice of housing noisy patients together to function as an auditory "trial by mirror," shocking lunatics into quietude through the horror of confrontation with their own boisterous doubles. Yet in reality, psychiatrists acknowledged that "excitable cases tend to react on each other when closely associated" (Annual Report 1910: 15). Patients housed in the violent wards and strong rooms of asylums tended to stay there, their symptoms aggravated rather than relieved by the noise of their fellow patients and the often brutalizing treatment of attendants.

By the late nineteenth century, psychiatrists acknowledged that, given the burgeoning population of patients, the "pernicious effects produced by the exposure of the quiet and sensitive" to the "noise of the other classes" could no longer "be avoided without radical departure from traditional hospital plans" (Bancroft 1889: 384). At Worcester, the accumulation of "noisy" patients was fed by the regulations of the Massachusetts State Board of Charities, which dealt with the overcrowding of asylums by transferring the more manageable and quiet insane to almshouses, leaving the asylum "wards filled with turbulent classes" (Annual Report 1909: 13). Rather than removing the noisy patients from the asylum—which was no longer an option given their overwhelming numbers—some psychiatrists suggested that the main hospital building be surrendered to the noisy, and the "reasonably quiet and orderly" patients given refuge in small, separate cottages (Annual Report 1895: 5). In the early 1870s, Worcester superintendent Dr. Merrick Bemis experimented with this plan, placing a small number of docile patients into a scattering of farmhouses on the hospital grounds. Bemis reported that these patients were "delighted by the removal from the noise and confusion of a great hospital" (Annual Report 1871: 9). However, the State Board was ultimately unwilling to abandon the familiar linear plan for what was still considered a radical deviation from standard hospital architecture.

LISTENING AS DIAGNOSTIC TOOL

Sound was used not only to classify patients en masse, organizing them on a population level but also to observe and diagnose the individual patient. The nineteenth century was an "age of 'auscultation,'" during which "physicians became virtuoso listeners" (Picker 2003: 6). Just as physicians might detect a defect in the heart or lungs by listening to them through a stethoscope (invented in 1816), psychiatrists claimed the ability to detect symptoms of mental illness through the vocalizations of the patient, translating the cacophony and incoherence of madness into legible signs. Through such practices of "codification," the *absence* of legible meaning—in the form of incomprehensible or irrational speech, or the absence of speech altogether—was suffused with signification in the form of diagnostic symptoms (Brian 2012: 313, 306). As psychiatrists claimed the ability to "hear" madness, as well as to see it, their ears were transfigured into instruments of observation and diagnosis (MacKinnon 2003: 75, 159). In doing so, they cultivated a particular "acoustemology," or "sonic way of knowing and being," founded on culturally informed ways of listening (Feld and Brenneis 2004: 426).

The efforts of psychiatrists to "read" the noise or silence of patients as symptoms had the inadvertent effect of divesting patients' actions of their intended meanings. Complaints about living conditions, requests for release, and allegations of abuse were all subsumed and silenced beneath the power they held as diagnostic signifiers. Accordingly, at the same time that psychiatrists' acoustemology primed them to receive certain types of information, they remained completely insensible to others (Camal 2019: 195). As Sally Swartz writes, "clinicians hear what their training enables them to hear," with the effect that "subaltern psychiatry maps both deafness and silence" (Swartz 2005: 507).

The distinctive patterns of "psychiatric audition" are evident in Pliny Earle's account of an unnamed male patient he treated while serving as the superintendent of the Bloomingdale Insane Asylum in New York in 1844 (Brian 2012). Earle described the man as a "negro whom I believe worthy of commemoration, for the purpose of showing how very insane, how abounding in delusions, and how incoherent a person may be," while retaining admirable "physical, intellectual, and moral" qualities. The meticulous recording of the patient's speech "in his own words" was undertaken for the sake of illustrating "his false ideas" and "incoherence." After recounting his history, former occupation, and family to Earle, the patient described his intentions to reorganize and remodel the Bloomingdale Asylum:

Patient.—I shall have a hundred nurses. I've seen them all; they're good looking people . . . I shall have four doctors. It's a very big house—will hold fifty thousand; that's the big part will hold so many. It has a steeple on it. The little part will hold a hundred; the next little part a hundred; the next fifty, the next forty; that's all. You may be one doctor if you've a mind to. We don't allow any man to sleep in the Asylum. We have a big hotel and bank. It's a little town, twenty-four miles round; a wall running round, twelve feet high, and more too, with iron pickets on the top, as big as your arm. The men will all sleep at the hotel.

I have a large farm and a large barn, fields, stables, peach orchard of twelve miles of peaches, two miles of cherries, ten miles of apples, twenty miles of pears; big pears, don't get ripe till very late—blue-bell pears, big round as your fist, most as big round as your head. There's a big blacksmith's shop, goldsmith's shop, and carpenter's shop; that's all the shops there is. There's a cabinet shop, but we don't use it; the man is dead that used to make bedsteads and bureaus. His name was Feenly; he died of the Cholera. He got sick in the morning, eating cabbage. He stole his wife's cabbage and eat it, and it killed him. He is buried in the Asylum; he's the only one buried there.

Physician.—Shall you use tranquilizing chairs and straps on your violent patients?

Patient.—No: nothing but the hard bed. Give them a hard room, nothing kept in it, and they never will do anything wrong again (Pliny Earle Papers 1844).While Earle recorded the patient's words as a symptom—the evidence of his insanity, just as a cough may be evidence of pneumonia—his description of a reimagined Bloomingdale may be viewed as a detailed critique of the asylum, revealing insight into what a patient thought the institution should and should not be, and addressed to the person (Earle) who held the most power to change it. Earle listened to the man as a patient, situating him within a specific and highly structured power dynamic; on the other hand, the patient spoke to Earle as his equal—that is, as one asylum administrator to another—thereby challenging the political structure of psychiatric audition as well as the material organization and therapeutic paradigm of the asylum.

This man was not the only patient at Bloomingdale with a plan to radically reconfigure the asylum. The case of B. H., age 33, was featured by Earle in the *American Journal of the Medical Sciences* in 1849 as a case of "partio-general paralysis." His methodical directives are worth quoting at length:

A canal is to commence at Hurlgate, and extend to the North Pole; and pass directly in front of this Asylum. All the waters in the world are to pass into it. All the commerce is to be carried through it by steamboats to be described here-after. The canal is to be four hundred feet wide, and twenty feet deep. The sides are to be laid with polished marble, and the bottom with free-stone taken from the Asylum building. The waters will have the sweetest perfumes, giving forth their odors only while the ladies promenade on its banks. All the fish and every thing that swims are to be gathered into these waters; but they will not hurt each other, owing to the fragrance of the waters. This seems to have an effect upon them similar to that of exhilarating gas upon man, only it continues as long as they remain in it.

The Asylum building is to be taken down, and a new one erected. The iron sashes are to be carried to the City, and made into printing presses to be in readiness for the new house, which is to be built of black marble, nine thousand and fifty stories high. This will bring it within fifty miles of heaven. Above this house, in the fifty miles mentioned, every twenty-five feet is to be a garden; this will make it high enough for any ornamental tree. In each of these gardens there is to be a spring, and the water is to have a very pleasant taste. They will all flow into one and form a fountain whose jet will rise many hundred feet . . . The different kinds of shrubbery are to be gathered from the ends of the earth, and arranged around the fountain according to their beauty.

The new house will accommodate billions of people. All the poor of Europe are to be brought over today and put into it, that they may be ready to go to a ball which he is to give to-night at Catskill. From the sale of the tickets he expects to make enough to pay for the house and furniture. The poor people are to be brought over by balloons, made so large that they can attach them to the houses, and bring them safe over with the people still in them.

We have a population of thirteen to a square mile: some states have only one: but when he gets the land covered with buildings made of rose-wood, golden floors, and every thing to correspond; with bedsteads of red cedar, so that there will be no bed bugs, the population will be very dense. The bed-rooms are to be elegantly furnished. Museums are to be established, and into them are to be gathered specimens of everything upon the face of the earth. Theatres are to be constructed in the most costly style. The birds are to be taught to sing by means of the hand-organ. The poor are to work one hour after each meal to give them exercise. The furniture of the present asylum is to be taken to the city and sold at auction. A painter is to be brought from France to-day, and all the painting of the new house is to be done by him tomorrow. The patients are to be cured by galvanism. All the land in this country is to be divided into farms of fifty acres each. (Pliny Earle Papers 1849)

The visions of the asylum conjured by these two patients are not simply evidence of their insanity. When read as treatises in their own right, each expresses its respective author's yearning for control over his surroundings. Each design is suffused with the idealistic confidence in the transformative power of the environment that was, at that time, beginning to fade from the psychiatric profession. Unencumbered by the austerity of state budgets and the limitations of medical science, they re-envision the asylum as the "utopia" that even W. A. F. Browne—writing at the height of therapeutic optimism— believed it could never be.

When juxtaposed against the realities of life in nineteenth-century asylums, these treatises appear all the more pointed in their critique. In response to the asylum's chronic staff shortages, the first man imagines a hundred "good looking" nurses. Both imagine that their asylums will hold a vast number of patients—"fifty thousand" or "billions": a vision that inverts the strained capacities of asylums faced with a rapidly increasing insane population. The "sweet perfumes" of the canal imagined by B. H. contrasts with the olfactory reality of the asylum (see chapter 3), while his visions of gold and black marble, rosewood, and golden floors speak to the characteristically bare and austere asylum interiors. Notably, Pliny Earle was renowned for being a particularly economical administrator. Following his tenure at Bloomingdale, he was hired as the superintendent of the Northampton State Hospital for the express purpose of checking its wasteful spending (Earle 1898: 263).

When B. H. imagines the iron sashes of the asylum being made into printing presses, he invokes the meaning with which patients vested these materials as emblems of their confinement, and the desire to remake them into instruments of expressivity. Perhaps most poignantly, the first man states that his asylum will not use mechanical restraint, or any form of discipline other than "a hard room." While a handful of mid-nineteenth-century American superintendents espoused the doctrine of "nonrestraint," Pliny Earle was not one of them. In an 1845 article in the *American Journal of Insanity*, he defended the use of the camisole (a type of straitjacket) at Bloomingdale as a "comfortable" form of restraint that "doesn't abrade [the] skin," comparing it favorably against the chains formerly used (Earle 1845: 8–9).

Notably, neither patient envisions the destruction of the asylum altogether; rather, he imagines an asylum remade in an image of luxury, abundance, and pleasure, stripped of all its discomforts and degradations. B. H., having invested in the asylum's promise of curability, identifies galvanism as the cure—a remarkably forward-thinking suggestion given that electricity was just beginning to be considered as a potential treatment for insanity. Pliny Earle, on the other hand, would go on to publish *The Curability of Insanity* (1877), a treatise that seriously undermined the reputation of asylums as curative institutions and suggested that insanity was not nearly as amenable to treatment as earlier psychiatrists had suggested. While the therapeutic paradigm was still ascendant in the 1840s, Earle was well aware that the disease with which he had diagnosed B. H. (general paralysis, first described by French psychiatrists only a few years earlier) had so far proven to be uniformly fatal ("Cases of paralysis peculiar to the insane" 1847). Whether he knew it or not, B. H.'s vision of being cured by galvanism stood at odds with the prognosis that Earle had given him.

That Earle was willing and able to record each man's speech in such detail, yet failed to view the resulting texts as anything but vocalized symptoms, is representative of the prevailing attitudes of nineteenth-century psychiatry. In writing that madness was "reduced to silence" by the machinations of the asylum (Foucault 1977: 250), Foucault failed to consider that patients were never silent; psychiatrists simply weren't listening. Yet the diagnostic apparatus constructed to capture patients' words as audible symptoms had the unintended effect of registering detailed expressions of criticism, imagination, and desire. Such expressions indicate that patients longed for a degree of control over the materiality of the asylum that even psychiatrists could not claim, and that they held out hopes for the cure that the asylum had promised, but had yet to deliver. Although these desires were swelled into grandiosity through the imaginative lens of their illness, they were still grounded in a keen awareness of the asylum's defects. Through the instruments of psychiatric audition, psychiatrists were capable of registering the grandiosity of their patients' statements while remaining deaf to their critical insights.

The "deafness" of psychiatric audition would have been particularly pronounced in cases where psychiatrists were literally unable to understand their patients' speech. Non-English-speaking immigrants represented an increasingly large proportion of asylum inmates over the course of the nineteenth century. Negative stereotypes linking immigrants with immorality, vice, and disease colored psychiatrists' perceptions of their patients' sanity. In order to better "enact the part of a poor, unfortunate crazy girl"—and thus gain admission to an insane asylum—Nellie Bly peppered her answers to police officers' questions with bits of Spanish and told a judge that she was from Cuba (Bly 1887). The suggestion of foreign nativity gave credence to Bly's performance as a lunatic. Once confined, Bly discovered that many of her fellow inmates were immigrants whose fates were determined by doctors wholly unable to understand them. Bly describes the half-hearted attempt of a physician to communicate with a German-speaking patient through the aid of a nurse who, while of German ancestry, "could understand but few words of her mother tongue." According to Bly, the German patient was thus "consigned to the asylum without a chance of making herself understood" (ibid.). Woodward believed that "we are not so successful in our treatment of [immigrants] as with the native population of New England," a fact he attributed partly to failures in communication (Annual Report 1847: 33). Notably, he placed the blame for these failures not on the physician's inability to understand or secure an interpreter, but to immigrants' "embarrassment from not clearly understanding our language" (ibid.).

In the early twentieth century, the skill of listening assumed new currency in the psychiatric profession. Mobilizing the physiology of Helmholtz as a metaphor for psychoanalysis, Freud stated that the psychiatrist must "act as a sympathetic resonator; a device to reconstitute and clarify the unconscious that emerges in vocal communication with the present" (Picker 2003: 108). Yet Freud, like Earle, conceived the process of listening to the patient not as a means of hearing what the patient was saying, but of recovering the *hidden* symbology embedded in the patient's discourse. To Earle, this was speech as symptom; to Freud, it was speech as a channel to the subconscious, a source of meaning that was inaccessible to the patient and might even directly contradict the literal substance of what he or she said. In both cases, the content of the patient's discourse was glossed over, his speech conceived as a series of coded messages that only the psychiatrist could decipher. In this quest to recover "true" meaning—that is, the meaning that mattered to psychiatrists—the patient's actual words were ignored. Accordingly, while Freud's "talking cure" marks a major development in the history of psychiatric audition, the "story of the rise of listening" in psychiatry is also one of the profession's continuing deafness—or more accurately, refusal to listen (ibid.: 87).

SOUND AS THERAPY

As a complementary strategy to eliminating the negative influences posed by pathological noise, psychiatrists mobilized therapeutic forms of sound as a positive influence on patients ("Case of mental excitement allayed by music" 1846, Zeller 1850: 200). The wards of the first Worcester State Hospital resounded with the serenades of visiting musicians, ensembles of patients playing various instruments, and in February 1851, a troupe of Swiss bell ringers (Annual Report 1851: 60). The "better" wards were furnished with pianofortes, which were used to accompany dances in the winter balls, and cages of singing birds to simulate the calming scenes of nature (Annual Report 1848: 53.). Music was believed to act upon patients' nervous system through the affective states it inspired: "according to its quality music has an animating or lulling effect upon the invalid listener; gives courage to the patient, [and] fills the convalescent with joyous hope of a speedy restoration" (Blumer 1892: 353).

The first hospital chapel, built in 1837, provided a setting for the singing of hymns. A choir composed of patients and attendants was formed that year, and by 1843, consisted of twenty to thirty members with two to four musical instruments (Annual Report 1837: 8, 1843: 86). By invoking themes such as the "light" of reason and the "darkness" of mental illness, the hymns sung by the choir formalized associations between morality, medical treatment, and sensory experience. Woodward believed that "sacred music is one of the safest and most salutary exercises for the insane," and claimed that "those who are often greatly excited, restless and noisy in the halls" were quiet in the chapel (Annual Report 1841: 86, 1840: 84). Balls and dances had a similar effect. As described to a local newspaper by an anonymous patient in October 1836, a special event at the hospital concluded with "a march . . . which moved all, and quelled or quieted those whom the more lively airs had affected; after marching a few moments, they were all seated and entertained, and then all happily conducted to their respective chambers" ("Scene at an insane hospital" 1836). At the hospital's 1836 Thanksgiving celebration (also described by an anonymous patient in a newspaper account) "the effect [of the music] was immediate, and it was interesting to see [the patients] one after another arise from their seats, unrequested and unmolested, and very cheerily with noiseless feet (for I observed they had slipped off [their] shoes), glide down the long hall and seem to feel themselves unfettered, free, quite regardless of all around them" ("Scene at an insane hospital" 1836).

Musical events at Worcester and other insane hospitals were said to have a tranquilizing, normalizing, and leveling effect on patients; their symptoms temporarily alleviated, "freed" from the binds of mental illness and the weight of confinement, patients were able to engage with each other, the attendants and physicians of the asylum, and even the superintendent and his family as dance partners and social actors. Woodward, his wife, and children all danced with the patients at these events as one large "family." During his tour of England in 1860, Edward Jarvis attended a ball at the Lunatic Asylum in Powick, during which the assistant physician played the piano and Jarvis danced with several patients. According to Jarvis, the patients at the ball were indistinguishable from sane dancers in "their motions, their intermingling, their performance of their respective parts, their steps & connection with the music" (Jarvis 1860). He heartily endorsed the use of music and dancing "to keep the patients' minds and bodies in sane action." Notably, these events and the weekly chapel service were the only times that male and female patients were able to interact with—or even see—each other.

Descriptions of the effects of music on asylum patients verged on the miraculous, with psychiatrists even comparing it to David's use of the harp to drive out evil spirits from Saul in the Old Testament (Blumer 1892: 359): an allusion that speaks to the premodern notion of mental illness as demoniacal possession. Yet these psychiatrists were sure to secure the use of music within the biomedical model by articulating its action in terms of the connection between sensory experience, mind, and body, and by contextualizing it within the genealogy of ancient medical treatises, including those of Herodotus and Pausanias, who recognized the ability of music to "civilize men" (Esquirol 1845: 80). Because music was said to act "directly" on the mind, "without the intervention of the consciousness of the individual upon the internal motor impulses," it was considered to be a more powerful tonic than those whose machinations were obvious to the patient ("The mental operations in health and disease" 1866: 300). Like the optical tricks of the asylum described in chapter 2, the efficacy of the hospital's hypnotic melodies was dependent on the mystified nature of their action.

Some psychiatrists may have held out the hope that their patients might be miraculously cured by music, as in the case reported in the *Illinois & Indiana Medical & Surgical Journal* in 1846:

> A violin player was sent for, and the effect of his art tested upon the patient, with the most remarkable and immediate favorable effects. The nervous excitement began to abate at the sound of the fiddle, and in a very short time, the patient was in a sound sleep, from which he awoke in an hour or two much refreshed and nearly rational. ("Case of mental excitement allayed by music" 1846: 149–150)

However, for the most part, music was seen as a way of calming, subduing, and entertaining the insane, and not as a direct means of curing them (Blumer 1892). In the words of Etienne Esquirol, music may "bring peace and composure, but [it] does not cure" (Esquirol 1845: 80).

Furthermore, psychiatrists took for granted that what they perceived as pleasant or unpleasant sounds would be perceived in the same manner by patients suffering from severe mental illness. Yet while he was debilitated by catatonic depression, Clifford Beers perceived the hymns he heard drifting from the hospital chapel as "funeral dirges" (Beers 1913: 14). It was only months later that Beers perceived the reading of a particular psalm in the chapel as a positive sign, signaling great promise and potential—yet, as he writes, this optimism was only an early symptom of his transition from a depressive to a manic state, in which he perceived encouraging messages and instructions embedded in his surroundings. Beers's account suggests that a patient's affective polarity—particularly when pushed to the extreme ends of the emotional spectrum—could play a large part in determining whether a sound would be interpreted as positive or negative, threatening or full of hope. While psychiatrists intended the environment to mold mental illness, in such cases, mental illness molded the environment into a reality that was specific to the patient.

Much like the bucolic landscapes and pleasantly furnished interiors initially constructed for the asylum, the harmonious soundscapes of the asylum tended to deteriorate over time, under the ravages of neglect. The chapel fell into disrepair; overcrowding meant that the halls constantly brimmed with noise, and events involving the entire asylum population became increasingly infeasible. One incident from her ten days at the Blackwell's Island Asylum recounted by Nellie Bly serves as a poignant representation of the deterioration of the therapeutic asylum, both literally and figuratively. Entreated by the nurses to play the piano that was stationed in the ward, Bly "struck a few notes, and the untuned response sent a grinding chill through me" (Bly 1887).

"AN AMAZING CHORUS OF SCREAMS"

As discussed in chapter 1, the removal of lunatics from society served a dual purpose in relieving them from pathological environments and in relieving the sane from interaction with the insane. In discussing the siting of the asylum, psychiatrists acknowledged that the inhabitants of cities would be "annoyed by the noise and sight of the violent" (Falret 1854: 225). However, they failed to anticipate the impressive cacophony of sounds that would be produced by congregating large numbers of the insane in a single building, regardless of how well classified they were. Elizabeth R. Hill described the noise of other patients in the Worcester State Hospital as "more torturing than a scorpion's whip" (Hill 1881: 26, 34). "I begged them to give me a room where I might not hear the talk or see the insane," she wrote. Nonetheless, in her room "the head radiators brought the most loathsome, profane, incoherent yells and shrieks around that could be made by the most raven lost minds." She lamented, "Oh, could I secure an atmosphere of quiet from this maniac rabble!" (ibid.).

Beers gave a similar description of the soundscape of the violent ward to which he was committed in 1905:

> The short corridor in which I was placed was known as the "Bull Pen" . . . it was usually in an uproar . . . Patients in a state of excitement may sleep during the first hours of the night, but seldom all night; and even should one have the

capacity to do so, his companions in durance would wake him with a shout or a song or a curse or a kicking of a door. A noisy and chaotic medley frequently continued without interruption for hours at a time. Noise, unearthly noise, was the poetic license allowed the occupants of these cells . . . I question whether I averaged more than two or three hours sleep a night during that time. (Beers 1913: 70)

According to Beers, the din of the violent ward was contagious. In order to command attention, he "learned to be more noisy than my neighbors," despite the fact that such "demonstrations" often led to violent abuse by the attendants.

Faced with the "terrible shrieks which came from all directions" in the Jacksonville Asylum, Mrs. Olsen, a patient and friend of Elizabeth Packard, "stuff[ed] cotton into my ears to deaden the sounds," but did not experience relief. The noise gave her such a severe headache that she feared she would go insane, corroborating Packard's assertion that the environment of an asylum could drive a sane person out of her mind. To soothe herself, Olsen figured out how to "neutralize the effect of such sounds by reversing the current of their ideas . . . Sitting up, erect in my bed, with as loud a voice as I could possibly command, to help drown these opposite voices, I repeated passages of the most beautiful and attractive poetry I had ever learned in former years" (Packard 1873: 313). In its capacity to direct her patterns of thought into more positive channels through repetitious behavior, Olsen's strategy was less like the environmental approach of moral treatment and more like modern cognitive behavioral therapy. In enabling her to separate from her environment, this strategy allowed her to construct her own "asylum"—a true sanctuary—in her mind. Packard claimed that her faith served a similar purpose in allowing her to build a refuge within herself during her confinement. Such practices suggest the ability of patients to build "quiet havens" within themselves, constructed of mental and spiritual habits, intended to insulate them against the pernicious influences of the brick-and-mortar asylum.

Patients attested that they were distressed not only by the noise of other patients but also by the distinctive and often unremitting auditory cues of confinement. Robert Fuller wrote that "the ringing of bells, the doors grating on their hinges, and the groans of the distressed—all combined to shed an air of gloom over my apartment" during his first night at McLean, to the extent that he was unable to sleep (Fuller 1833: 14). Nellie Bly described a similar racket on the first night of her stay in the insane ward of Bellevue Hospital, consisting of the sirens of approaching ambulances, screams from the men's ward, and the sound of nurses continuously talking and "walk[ing] heavily down the halls, their boot-heels resounding like the march of a private of dragoons" (Bly 1887). Conolly recognized that "the jingling of keys, the clang of locks, and the violent opening and shutting of doors produce uncomfortable feelings in patients" (Conolly 1847: 32). Following this advisory, the administrators of the Wakefield Asylum in England chose to "eliminat[e] [the] grating sounds made by bolts on patient doors" by substituting mortice locks (Cherry 1989: 142). At Conolly's own asylum at Hanwell, attendants patrolling the wards at night were instructed to wear "cloth shoes" to avoid disturbing sleeping patients (Conolly 1847: 102).

Nonetheless, psychiatrists could not eliminate all of the sounds that defined the soundscape of the asylum and distinguished it from the environments from which patients had been removed. Rather than finding the asylum a "quiet haven," patients found it to be a chorus of strange, unfamiliar, and distressing sounds that served to constantly remind them of their confinement. Patients were not the only residents of the asylum who found its soundscape to be unpleasant and unnerving. Among the complaints lodged during the 1902 nurses' strike at the Worcester State Hospital was the fact that attendants' rooms were located on the same floor as the patients, so that staff were subjected to constant "shrieks and screams in the night" (*Worcester Telegram* 1902). Although attendants were technically free to leave, their long hours, low pay, and lack of viable employment alternatives meant that many felt themselves virtually indentured by the asylum, a reality that was belabored by their inability to escape the auditory presence of insanity even while trying to sleep.

"QUIETING" AS RESTRAINT

Many of the methods for "treating" mental illness, both before and after the creation of the therapeutic asylum, were targeted at eliminating or lessening the distinctive symptoms of insanity. Sound and fury were foremost among the symptoms that physicians intended to alleviate. In the period preceding the opening of the Worcester State Hospital, bloodletting was frequently used in the treatment of insane people in their homes, in particular to lessen the agitation of mania (Rush 1830). While Woodward wrote in the hospital's 1841 annual report that bleeding was "no longer considered a viable *treatment*" for insanity (emphasis added), it continued to be used to provide "temporary relief" from manic symptoms and to "subdue" the noisy and intractable patient (Annual Report 1844: 70–71). In 1844, Woodward described the case of a patient who was bled extensively while in the asylum, reporting that "all efforts failed of curing his insanity (though he is quieter)" (ibid.). By 1854, Pliny Earle acknowledged that venesection was numbered among the instruments in the psychiatrists' toolkit that could not be considered cures or even treatments for insanity, but had the desired effect of quieting manic patients, thereby rendering them more amenable to the machinations of the asylum (Earle 1854: 15).

Nineteenth-century psychiatrists prided themselves in abandoning or minimizing the use of the methods used to control insanity by previous generations, including "heroic" treatments such as bloodletting and purging, and the use of mechanical restraint. In their place, psychiatrists developed an arsenal of strategies that might be considered "passive" restraints, which produced the same tranquilizing effects as earlier, "barbaric" methods, but were perceived as gentle, humane, and scientific. Like Willis's overpowering "EYE," the psychiatrist's voice constituted one of the earliest instruments identified as indirect means of controlling the insane patient (Rush 1830: 175). Similarly, music functioned as a type of "sonic straitjacket" or "aestheticized restraint" (MacKinnon 2003: 160). Patients were exposed to "the open air" out of a belief that it was "of its own nature, *calming*" (Parigot 1863: 401, emphasis original). They were subjected to labor in order to make them too tired to produce "mischief and noise" (Annual Report 1840: 75). At the Worcester State Hospital, a generous diet was served because Woodward believed that "insane persons usually sleep better at night after full suppers" (Woodward Papers n.d.). Writing to Pliny Earle, Dr. H. B. Wilbur, superintendent of the New York State Hospital at Syracuse, refuted allegations that British asylums were only able to dispense with mechanical restraint by substituting the use of narcotics. He found instead that "[t]he occupation of patients, the employment of night attendants and improved diet & regimen are obviating the necessity for any kind of restraint" (Wilbur 1879). Similarly, Dr. J. Leslie Tobey stated that "plenty of fresh air, good food, abundant exercise and pleasant surroundings are better than chloral" in subduing patients ("Proceedings of the association" 1891: 89).

Passive restraint was not only targeted at controlling patients but in also making them more amenable to or less aware of that control and therefore less likely to contest it. In the *American Journal of Insanity,* G. Alder Blumer of the Utica State Hospital suggested the use of music to regulate labor in the asylum, pointing out that "in the South, negroes perform appointed tasks with greater patience by reason of the inspiriting effect of their rollicking melodies" (Blumer 1892). That such practices developed partly as a means to weather the hardship of labor under slavery is a fact that Blumer does not acknowledge, but the implicit connection is there: like slaves, asylum patients were confined against their will and labored without payment. Although psychiatrists resented both the comparison between asylums and the heavily stigmatized institutions of slavery and imprisonment, their use of segregation and isolation to control "noisy" patients was partly an inheritance of the Pennsylvania System, a method of prison discipline developed at the Eastern State Penitentiary in the early nineteenth century ("Notices of books" 1845:

381). Quaker reformers believed that the enforced silence and seclusion of the Pennsylvania System would engender the same effect as their silent religious meetings, during which individuals were suffused with the Inner Light; the "light" that was intended to reach prisoners was both spiritual and moral, and culminated in the achievement of penitence. Although the rules and regulations of the asylum as written were not this extreme, in practice patients who were confined to solitary cells lived under conditions that were just as austere as any prison that practiced the Pennsylvania System. Furthermore, although the disciplinary methods used at the asylum were couched in terms of "treatment," patient accounts indicate that they were often perceived as punitive and cruel, as bad if not worse than the tactics used against slaves and prisoners.

When the more "modern" strategies of passive restraint and solitary confinement failed, psychiatrists resorted to more direct means to subdue patients and thereby reassert their dominance over the asylum soundscape. While English and Scottish asylums followed (or claimed to follow) the doctrine of "nonrestraint," American superintendents endorsed the use of the camisole, the muff, the straitjacket, and other means of mechanical restraint. Chemical restraint—in the form of narcotic drugs—was also regularly used to subdue noisy patients. Morphine was said to render patients "more quiet, rational, and natural" (Annual Report 1844: 74), while chloral hydrate was "efficacious in quieting habitually noisy patients at night" ("Proceedings of the association" 1876: 276). Woodward made liberal use of conium, belladonna, and opium in his treatment of mental disorders both at the Worcester State Hospital and in his private practice. In "cases of high excitement," he recommended the application of "nauseating doses of emetics," in addition to narcotics, to "produce quiet and composure" (Woodward Papers n.d.).

Many patients were distrustful of medicines and often resisted taking them, fearing that they might be sickened, killed, or driven insane. Elizabeth Stone believed that the medicine given to her while she was a patient at McLean "harden[ed] or petrifie[d]" the part of her brain governing love and affection, rendering her incapable of happiness (Stone 1842). Bly reported that the nurses at Blackwell's Island Asylum "inject so much morphine and chloral that the patients are made crazy. I have seen the patients wild for water from the effect of the drugs, and the nurses would refuse to give it to them" (Bly 1887). Packard described a fellow patient at the Jacksonville Asylum, Mrs. Cheneworth, who was given opium "as a quietus to her then excited nervous system" (Packard 1873: 232–233). When Cheneworth's condition deteriorated, culminating in her suicide, Packard described her as "a victim to that absurd practice of the medical profession, which depends upon poisons instead of nature to cure disease" (ibid.).

Patients were not the only ones who believed that the use of sedating medicines in the asylum was dangerous and even potentially lethal. In 1865, testimony concerning the case of Charles Frost, a twenty-eight-year-old man whose death at the Boston Lunatic Hospital was attributed by his family to the improper use of ether, was heard before the city government (Ellis 1866). A decade later, a report attributing a series of patient deaths in asylums to the use of chloral provoked controversy and debate among American psychiatrists ("Proceedings of the association" 1876: 275–277). In response, a resolution was proposed at the annual meeting of the AMSAII stipulating "that chloral should be employed with great caution, [and] only on the prescription of a reputable physician" ("Proceedings of the association" 1876: 275). Calling the resolution "superfluous," Dr. Alexander E. MacDonald refuted the association of patient deaths with chloral and stated that the danger was overestimated, citing his own liberal use of the drug at the New York City Asylum for the Insane at Ward's Island, without "untoward results" (ibid.). The debate was still active at the annual meeting in 1891, when Dr. C. H. Hughes decried what he viewed as the "overuse of hypnotics" in asylums, suggesting that psychiatrists used them "for the sole purpose of suppressing every sort of abnormal cerebral manifestation," and stating that "chemical suppression of symptoms is not the cure of disease" ("Proceedings of the association" 1891: 88–89). On this last point, at least, psychiatrists could agree. They recognized that the medicines used to quiet the insane, like music, were "convenient and useful, but have no curative power" (Earle 1877: 530).

When sanctioned methods of quieting patients failed, asylum attendants substituted others in their place. Some of these strategies were violent: Beers reported that attendants faced with a "noisy patient" "kicked or choked [him] into a state of temporary quiet" (Beers 1913: 70), while Bly reported witnessing a "hysterical" patient "choked" and "dragged" until "I heard her terrified cries hush into smothered ones" (Bly 1887). The threat of violence was effective in quieting even "normal" forms of speech. When asked why they didn't tell the superintendent "how they were suffering from the cold and insufficiency of clothing" when he came to visit them, Bly's fellow patients informed her that "the nurse would beat them if they told" (ibid.). Attendants also cultivated their own passive or indirect means of controlling patients. One attendant, faced with Clifford Beers' incessant talking during his manic state, managed to trick him into a day-long silence by telling Beers he "was so crazy [he] could not possibly keep [his] mouth shut for even one minute" (Beers 1913: 66–67). Accordingly, in some instances, the relative quiet of the wards may have had less to do with the efficacy of the asylum in calming patients' nerves and more to do with the tactics of intimidation and persuasion used by attendants.

SOUND AS DOMINATION AND RESISTANCE

An effective asylum functioned much like a factory in its ability to marshal large amounts of human biopower into a mechanized system of production, and in its use of ideology to shape individuals' behavior and identities (Annual Report 1881: 16). The asylum as "moral machinery" thus produced both people and products, mobilizing the productivity of labor itself as a means to convert lunatics into docile workers (Skålevåg 2002: 55). Psychiatrists acknowledged that asylums were "factory like" in their architectural style and monumentality (Bell 1845: 16). In some cases, this resemblance was intentionally cultivated by psychiatrists and state commissioners who consulted factory architects on the best means of building a large state hospital ("Proceedings of the association" 1884: 81–82). Although unpaid, patients who were put to work at the asylum labored in ways that were similar to their sane counterparts in the industrializing city. The bell system functioned in the same way at the Worcester State Hospital as it would have at the nearby factories, as a source of auditory cues to reinforce control and regulate the management of time. The sound of the bell routed itself in a Pavlovian manner into the patient's mind and body, becoming an agent in the institution's function to instill discipline, dividing and reifying time into easily quantifiable segments (Leone and Potter 1999: 202).

While the bell system was considered indispensable to the asylum's ability to function as a productive entity, many patients found its insistent noise distressing. In 1879, A. P. Reid, superintendent of the Nova Scotia Hospital for the Insane, reported his experiments with an alternative "means of communicating with different parts of the institution," citing the inconvenience of electric bells that were "apt to be out of order" and could "only communicate in one direction" ("Proceedings of the association" 1879: 218). The "speaking tubes" that Reid designed using old steam coils were intended to allow verbal messages to be sent up to 500 feet across the asylum. Because "a slight tap of a key is heard with great distinctness the whole length of the line," Morse code could also be substituted for speech. At the Worcester State Hospital, however, the electric bell system was supplanted only by the radio, which allowed physicians to be paged across the asylum. Administrators reported that "hallucinated [*sic*] patients show less agitation at paging than bells" (Annual Report 1938: 39). At the same time that this transition took place, administrators made an effort to downplay the factory-like aspect of the asylum, refashioning patient labor into "occupational therapy."

The function of the asylum to control patients by selectively amplifying and muffling sound was contested by patients' continual efforts to upset the institutional balance between noise and quiet. While interpreted by psychiatrists chiefly as a symptom of insanity, patients' noisiness can also be seen as part of a "constellation of everyday activities intended to undermine, thwart, or obstruct conditions of domination" (Casella 2009: 24). Beers wrote that the noisy "demonstrations" he performed during his confinement in the violent ward "were partly in fun and partly by way of protest" (Beers 1913: 70). Unable to control their own movements or the nature of their environment, "[m]aking noise was one of the only means of resistance open to patients," and their cacophonies overwhelmed all efforts on the part of psychiatrists to control the soundscape of the asylum (Fennelly 2014: 427). Noise was one of the few acts of resistance in which patients could be said to have "collaborated." Despite psychiatrists' beliefs that the insane were rendered cripplingly self-absorbed by their illness and thus unable to work with each other in any meaningful way, patients did cooperate in the creation of the asylum soundscape, raising their voices together and over one another's, as Beers described.

The asylum instituted a variety of strategies aimed at subduing or silencing patient voices, particularly those that threatened the sanctity of the asylum order. These voices were not only corporeal but include those encoded in written messages. Patient letters and accounts served as one important mode of subverting the enforced silences of the asylum. In most asylums, psychiatrists held the power to read patients' letters and to prevent them from being sent to their intended recipients if they believed it to be in the patients' best interest ("Proceedings of the association" 1872: 243; Hrdlička 1899: 402). Packard describes how superintendent McFarland confiscated both her letters and her writing implements in an attempt to stop her protests from reaching the outside world. In response, Packard secreted her journal, in which she recorded her testimony of life in the Jacksonville Asylum, in between the glass and the backboard or her mirror and behind a false lining in her bandbox (Packard 1873). She wrote on tissue paper and in the margins of newspapers. Permitted to embroider pieces of clothing to be sent to her daughters, she wrote messages to them on the fabric. Lydia Denny threw her letters onto the road during the carriage rides outside of the McLean Asylum, hoping that they would be found and delivered to her friends (Denny 1862). "Never allowed pen, ink, [or] paper," she wrote with "bits of pencil, saved paper from parcels, [and] blank leafs from books."

The contents of patients' letters, like their vocalized messages, were seen primarily as expressions of symptoms by nineteenth-century psychiatrists (Annual Report 1844: 93), and are read in the same way by twenty-first-century clinicians. Allan Beveridge, a medical historian and psychiatrist at the University of Glasgow, writes that the sample of nineteenth-century patient letters preserved at the Royal Edinburgh Asylum demonstrates the "unchanging nature of mental illness" (Beveridge 1997: 907). Like their counterparts today, he writes, the mentally ill individuals at the asylum displayed "delusions of control." Yet because the asylum was an institution primarily aimed at transforming the lunatic into a sane person by manipulating his senses, patients' perceptions that they were being controlled were, in fact, an accurate reflection of their situation. Like Pliny Earle's patients, described above, these patients may have suffered from mental illness, but the fact of their insanity does not mean that their judgments of the asylum were incorrect. On the contrary, through their ability to imagine alternative realities in which the privations and horrors of the asylum were mitigated by luxury and freedom, patients proved themselves capable of seeing the asylum for what it really was: a site of confinement, control, and contested power, whose therapeutic promise was undercut by its material limitations.

CONCLUSION: SOUND AND SUBJECTIVITY

While psychiatrists distinguished between "good" sounds and "bad" sounds as though these constituted objective categories, they failed to consider the possibility that sounds of any type might be interpreted in a myriad of ways—both good and bad—by a person suffering from insanity. Beers described how "the most trifling occurrence"—namely, the sound of ice clinking against the side of a pitcher of water—assumed "vast significance" when refracted through the lens of his illness. Haunted by delusions that he was being pursued by law enforcement, he believed that the sound "was produced by some mechanical device resorted to by the detectives for a purpose" (Beers 1913). Similarly, he believed that the sound of a thunderstorm was "man-made . . . due to some clever contrivance of my persecutors," while the sound of the electric bell in the asylum used to summon attendants provoked "a mild shock of terror, for I imagined that at last the hour had struck for my transportation to the scene of trial" (ibid.: 14, 35).

Beers's experience was representative of his own unique "sonic persona": a term Jerome Camal uses to describe the embodiment of "idiosyncratic modes of sensory engagement with the world" that "form the basis of individual subjectivity" (Camal 2019: 195). Nineteenth-century psychiatrists failed to appreciate that the asylum was not the only force that was shaping patients' sonic personae. Mental illness also played sensory tricks on patients, transmuting what was believed to be objectively pleasant stimuli into negative ones, and warping seemingly benign therapeutic strategies into instruments of torture. Additionally, the experience of confinement itself lent a negative cast to pleasant scenes, even in those patients who did not suffer from mental illness, such as Elizabeth Packard and Nellie Bly. Patients who believed they were being imprisoned or persecuted were almost always viewed as delusional by psychiatrists. Yet the reality of the asylum's efforts to confine and control patients gives credence to the conspiratorial interpretation of patients.

Psychiatrists' unwillingness to recognize and accommodate the subjectivities of their patients undermined their therapeutic endeavor. The asylum represented their efforts to construct a singular type of experience, a world that would be perceived by patients just as it was intended by its architects. Such a construction took for granted that one person's experience was the same as another's. The asylum was not one world, but an infinity of different worlds populated by the respective inhabitants of various subjective points of view. Accordingly, patients' perceptions of their experience in the asylum were as valid as any other, and despite—or perhaps because of—the distorting lens of their mental illness, they represented some of the most discerning and pointed critics of the asylum.

Chapter 4

The Smell of the Insane

Disciplining the Olfactory Domain

Like the visual and the auditory domains, the olfactory was claimed as an avenue for intervention into the insane mind by nineteenth-century psychiatrists, who argued that insanity had proliferated and worsened partly due to the noxious odors of the environments in which modern people lived. In the decades preceding the construction of the first lunatic hospitals, mental health reformers depicted the typical living conditions of the pauper insane as incompatible with health and well-being, appealing to their audience's visceral disgust toward filth and its attendant odors. The vivid and horrifying descriptions of pauper lunatics "confined . . . in *cages, closets, cellars, stalls, pens! Chained, naked, beaten with rods,* and *lashed* into obedience!" disseminated in the treatises of asylum reformer Dorothea Lynde Dix, a devoted ally of the Worcester State Hospital, helped to galvanize public support for the asylum movement across the United States, beginning in her home state of Massachusetts, where she documented the "*foul* spectacle" of "increasing accumulations of filth" and "offensive" air in pauper lunatics' accommodations (Dix 1843).

Exposure to vitiated air was considered not only unpleasant but also a serious health hazard. Prior to the discovery and dissemination of germ theory, miasmas—clouds of polluted gases exuded from pollution and waste—were thought to be responsible for the spread of infectious disease. A supply of clean and constantly replenished air was considered essential to health; "without it, [the lungs] are starved and the blood poisoned" (Black 1873: 34). Prior to industrialization, it was not difficult to meet this need. However, with the construction of cities, human beings were corralled into tight spaces, where they were suffocated by air pollution. Even the home could not provide a reprieve, as domestic spaces contained a noxious mix of "matters exhaled from the body, gas-lights and lamps, unclean floors and bedding, artificial impurities, [and] decomposing organic matter" (Black 1873: 51–52).

Given these insalubrious conditions, it was unsurprising that the inhabitants of cities were reported to suffer from diseases, including insanity, at alarming rates. Furthermore, it was believed that "the diseased and disturbed organization of lunatics is acutely sensitive to atmospheric influences" (Inspectors of Prisons 1849: 14). Accordingly, the asylum aimed at removing the insane from these conditions and immersing them in the pure atmosphere of country life. This endeavor was not unique to the asylum, but represented part of the larger process whereby "[m]odernity declared war on smells" (Bauman 1993: 24). As Zygmunt Bauman writes, odors were threatening not only to sanitary and hygienic standards but also to moral and social order. Smells contradicted "everything modernity stood for," namely, "order, predictability, control, and self-control" (ibid.: 25). Accordingly, "scents had no room in the shiny temple of perfect order modernity set out to erect."

As an iconic temple of modernity, the asylum aimed at literally and metaphorically sanitizing the offensive aspects of the insane in order to meet bourgeois standards. The logic and mechanics through which this sanitization was carried out were entwined with those of colonialism, which aimed to "'civilize' the non-European 'other'" partly by "deodor[izing] that other" (Hamilakis 2014). As one early slogan of Unilever stated, "Soap is Civilization" (ibid.: 18). By virtue of their unpleasant and characteristic odors, which marked them as a deviation from the "fragrant" and "inodorate" elite, the insane were linked to other categories of difference, such as race, ethnicity, and class (Classen 1997: 409). Accordingly, the asylum was nested within parallel and overlapping projects to control deviant classes through their subjection to its "sensorial regime" (Hamilakis 2014).

However, because "scents are the most obstreperous, irregular, and defiantly ungovernable of all impressions," the administrators of the Worcester State Hospital faced what was perhaps their most challenging battle in mastering the olfactory domain of the asylum (Bauman 1993: 24). Like the architects of nineteenth-century cities, they failed to anticipate the hygienic challenges posed by the concentration of a large population under a single roof. In many instances, patients found themselves in accommodations that were as overcrowded and poorly ventilated as urban tenements. Under such conditions, the maintenance of pure air was virtually impossible. Although administrators worked to remedy these defects, their efforts persistently collided against the structural constraints imposed by the hospital's original builders, the financial restrictions imposed by the state, and the inherently Sisyphean task of maintaining an adequate level of hygiene in a congested and poorly designed building. While the opening of the second hospital in 1877 worked to remedy some of the defects of the first, the reprieve it provided was largely temporary. Throughout the nineteenth century and well into the twentieth century, the distinctive smell of confinement was identified by patients and staff as one of the most noticeable features of their experiences at the asylum, lingering in memory long after they had left. The "smellscape" of the asylum served to pin the embodied experience of odor to a particular place, "thus connecting self and surroundings in profound and transformative ways" (Jackson 2011: 606). While nineteenth-century psychiatrists tended to attribute the character of the asylum smellscape to difference—that is to the deviant and defective physiology of the insane—I argue in this chapter that, in fact, it was the olfactory signature of institutionalization, a tangible representation of the failure to achieve an orderly sensorial regime, which was brought about largely by psychiatrists' misdirected efforts to localize and target the disease in the individual, rather than in the system.

While previous chapters have focused on the dialectic between administrators—as the figures who were invested with the authority to craft and carry out the policies of the hospital—and patients, as the primary subjects of those policies, this chapter expands its focus to include that of hospital attendants and nurses: the rank-and-file of the hospital who were tasked with the implementation of policies, particularly those surrounding hygiene and hydrotherapy. The staff of the hospital played an essential role as the arbiters between the theory and practice of asylum therapeutics. Their roles often placed them in an untenable position: charged with the responsibility for fulfilling the administration's wishes, yet lacking the resources to do so, they were held personally accountable for many of the asylum's failures. Many patient accounts describe how attendants perverted the therapeutic methods of the asylum into modes of physical and mental torture. While such actions were inexcusable, they cannot be easily rationalized away by pinning blame solely on the cruelty of individual attendants. The consistency of abusive actions—as well as the persistence of subpar living conditions—suggests the influence of systemic factors in making the olfactory domain of the asylum into a site of neglect, misery, and terror. In order to understand these systemic factors, it is necessary to analyze the role of attendants in negotiating between the top-down authority of administrators and the vulnerable population of asylum patients.

VENTILATION

One of the first and most persistent endeavors of the architects of the Worcester State Hospital was to ensure that the building was equipped with a functioning apparatus for ventilation so that its air would be constantly purified. Accordingly, the asylum was designed with furnaces in the basement, providing "a large column of pure air from out of doors," which was forced through the halls and rooms of the asylum and exited through flues in the walls, which in turn opened into skylights and windows in the attic (Annual Report 1836: 22, 1838: 72, 1841: 78). While this system was lauded as technologically advanced at the time the hospital opened in 1833, within two decades it had been rendered largely obsolete. By 1853, administrators complained that the "furnaces in the basement are nearly worn out," that they easily caught fire, and that "their ventilation is so imperfect as not to deserve the name . . . But for the natural ventilation through windows and doors, the contaminated air would often be intolerable" (Annual Report 1853: 13–14). Administrators attributed the preponderance of the skin infection erysipelas among patients to their exposure to the polluted air of the hospital (ibid.). Although it is now known that erysipelas is caused by the bacterium *Streptococcus*, administrators' perception that the environment played a role in its proliferation was probably correct, as the crowded conditions, close confinement, and inadequate hygiene in the hospital likely contributed to its spread among patients.

From the mid-nineteenth century onward, records of the trustees' visits to the hospital are populated by a near constant stream of complaints about the "noxious odors" that proliferated within its walls. Trustees noted the disjuncture between different sensory experiences of the hospital, namely sight and smell, stating that although "[t]o the *eye* all was neat, orderly, and seemly; to the smell, much was offensive, and even repulsive," indicating their frustration at failing to bring the various sensory regimes of the hospital into alignment (Trustees' Notes 1852). The trustees attributed the decline of the hospital's popular image partly to these "offensive" conditions. With improvements to its ventilating and heating mechanisms, they hoped "that the reputation of the Hospital will be sustained and its usefulness greatly increased" (Trustees' Notes 1854). These improvements came in the form of new steam furnaces and mechanical ventilators installed in the early 1850s. Along with the relocation of the water closets in the wings to keep their odors from saturating the halls, these changes were said to improve the air quality in the building.

Nonetheless, administrators' complaints continued over the next two decades, stating that the "arrangements for ventilation were never sufficient, [and] due to structural defects can never be made so" (Annual Report 1854: 34). The investigation by the Massachusetts State Commission of Lunacy led by Edward Jarvis in 1855 corroborated this finding, stating that the ventilation in the hospital was "very unsatisfactory," with the result that the air was "impure and insalubrious" (Jarvis 1855: 175, 180). Although modifications had been made to certain wings of the building with some benefit, the ventilation could not "be made satisfactory in other [wings] without a great and radical change in structure" (ibid.). The solidity with which the asylum had been built and the confidence of its architects in laying out what they perceived to be the ideal asylum plan made such crucial alterations difficult if not impossible. This fact made the abandonment of the building and its replacement by a newer model seem like the only solution. The construction of the second hospital, however, was still twenty years in the future. In the meantime, patients were forced to contend with the unsatisfactory living conditions in the hospital—and none suffered more than the inmates of the strong rooms.

STRONG ROOMS

The strong rooms or solitaries were not an original part of the construction of the Worcester State Hospital, but were added later to accommodate patients who were considered too violent for the wards ("Specifications of the additions . . . " 1835). The first were built in the mid-1830s. Within a few years, trustees regularly complained of their "dungeon-like aspect" and "foetid" air that was "disagreeable to breathe" (Trustees' Notes 1853). Unlike the apartments in the regular wards of the hospital, the strong rooms lacked windows—a violation of the architectural code laid out in almost every asylum treatise, as well as the official guidelines established by the AMSAII—and patients were often confined to them twenty-four hours a day, depriving them of many of the most important therapeutic resources of the asylum. The trustees wrote that the inhabitants of the strong rooms exhibited "shocking habits"—likely referring to the tendency of psychotic patients to smear their own excrement (Trustees' Notes 1854). Yet rather than attribute these behaviors solely to insanity, the trustees in this early period acknowledged that they were partly attributable to "the close confinement, & the vitiated air [that] lower the vital force, [which] beget a morbid condition of body, which of course beget a morbid condition of mind" (Trustees' Notes 1854).

Given their belief in the power of the environment to shape both mind and body, it is not surprising that the trustees believed that the conditions in the strong rooms—described below, in their own words—were sufficient to drive a sane man to insanity (all emphases original):

> In the solitaries of the South wing was noticed more offensive smells than I have observed before for a long time. The crowded state of the Hospital renders it necessary to occupy all those rooms and there is no cesspool so that everything offensive flows on the surface. It appeared to me that something ought to be done to relieve this evil (1841).

All the halls and apartments were found to be in usual good order, thoroughly clean and well ventilated, with the exception of the solitaries in the basement, which although properly cleaned, were offensive for the want of necessary ventilation (1846).

The weather was rainy and the air dense and close, and it was with exceeding gratification, that we found the Halls and Rooms clean and sweet, and the air, generally, and except in the lower tiers of the old strong rooms, fresh and pure (1849).

Every Room was visited, and with the Halls found perfectly clean and neat, and the air fresh and pure; unless the state of the old strong halls of the female department, always and necessarily from the want of better and other accommodations, occupied by the worst class of patients, who frequently defile themselves and their rooms in spite of all care; should be made an exception. The Patients seen in these Rooms, however, seemed as comfortable as the state of their malady should permit (1849).

The patients had nearly all risen and the windows has been partially opened. In most of the galleries and rooms the air was tolerably good and sweet, in others foul, demonstrating defective ventilation. The strong rooms in the northern wing on the basement floor were particularly foul. The ventilation of these rooms is so defective that they ought to be abandoned. (1851)

The strong rooms in the old part present the usual and striking offense to the senses which call so loudly for the abolishment of the[se?] dens[?] (1853).

The condition of several of the strong rooms, arising from the filthy habits of the inmates was such as to render them painful and disgusting (1853).

The patients in the strong room (strong to the smell as well as the touch) are as usual in a deplorable state. There can be no doubt that the rooms themselves – the cages or dens, rather, increase the irritability of the unfortunate creatures who are confined therein (1854).

A committee of the state legislature visiting the Worcester State Hospital in 1848 corroborated trustees' accounts, finding that the strong rooms had "the least advantages for light [and] none for ventilation," and were "unfavorably located, dark, dreary, damp & uncomfortable in that extent as to aggravate rather than to assist the cure of the unfortunate beings placed there" (Wyman 1877).

The terrible conditions of the strong rooms at Worcester were not unique. Complaints from both administrators and patients regarding the shockingly bad state of accommodations used to house violent patients in American asylums proliferated through the nineteenth and into the twentieth century. The padded cell occupied by Clifford Beers in 1905 was "a vile hole," suffering from a "lack of ventilation, which deficiency of course aggravates [its] general unsanitary condition" (Beers 1913: 63). The odor of the violent ward to which Elizabeth Packard was confined was so potent that it attached itself to its inmates, following them like an olfactory stigma wherever they went (Packard 1873: 116). Packard wrote that "[i]t is not possible for me to conceive of a more fetid smell, than the atmosphere of this hall exhaled."

Elizabeth R. Hill made similar complaints about the Worcester State Hospital, claiming that the blankets on her bed exuded a "sickening stench" that clung to her clothes. She attributed the smell to the fact that "a maniac [had] died on it" just before her arrival (Hill 1881: 34). "I have been told it was the rubber sheet," she wrote. Hill complained of the suffocating heat, and after "begg[ing] for a cooler room" she was moved to a cell that had also been occupied by a corpse "not one week before" (ibid.). Upon her release from the hospital, Hill wrote that she "felt the waters of Jordan, Abannar, and Parphar could not wash and soak out the stench that I had inhaled into my system" and the effects of "that terrible poisoning air" (ibid.: 44).

Following the principles of moral treatment, trustees were certain that if the patients in the strong rooms were placed in more healthful and home-like conditions, their behavior would improve. However, overcrowding and staff shortages forestalled such improvements until the construction of the second hospital. Even the architectural improvements provided by the new building did not completely mitigate the smells associated with the areas occupied by the hospital's most severely afflicted patients. The powerful odor of the violent wards may be partly attributed to defects in hospital design and partly to the inherent challenges of maintaining adequate hygiene in wards with incontinent and agitated patients. After two decades of experience, the trustees came to believe that "[n]ot all the brooms, scouring cloths, & whitewash brushes in the house, though kept in constant action, can <u>cleanse</u> a building like this one: in spite of the visible cleanliness, there is <u>smellible</u> dirt in many of the wards, & in all of the strong rooms" (Trustees' Notes 1853). While the "solid & tangible surface of things" may be cleaned, "when it comes to keeping the intangible atmosphere clean, it is impossible to succeed" (Trustees' Notes 1851).

This defeatist attitude toward conditions in the hospital was emblematic of the broader rise of pessimism that characterized the field of psychiatry beginning in the mid-nineteenth century. While the asylum had emerged as an institution aimed at healing the mind through mastering the physical senses, administrators had come to realize that "[s]mells ridicule the pretense of mastery" (Bauman 1993: 25). The odors of the asylum defied all attempts at discipline, turning the asylum into a battleground between chaos and order. By the late nineteenth century, psychiatrists had come to believe that chaos was winning. According to Andrew Scull, this is the period in which administrators "began to compromise and water down requirements, consoling themselves with the thought that the worst asylum was better than nothing" (Scull 1979:

113–114). Yet even this defeatism betrayed a stubborn confidence in the idea of the asylum itself, foreclosing all alternatives, even alternative models of asylums.[1] After all, to entertain alternatives to the asylum was to challenge the fundamental ideas behind the asylum, which were largely coterminous with the fundamental ideas of modernity. And so, even as the foundation of moral treatment seemed to collapse upon itself, nineteenth-century psychiatry never wavered in its faith in the asylum as the best solution to an intractable problem.

HYGIENE

Proper hygiene was widely espoused by physicians and health reformers in the nineteenth century as a prerequisite for good health. The natural functions of the body were thought to result in the creation of waste products that were secreted through the skin, where they combined with external pollutants to create a film of "gathered filth and accumulated excretions" (Jarvis 1845: 38). Without washing, this dirty coating would impede the natural respiration of the skin. To prevent the poisoning of the body by its own waste, health reformers advocated bathing at least once a week, exerting rigorous friction over the entire surface of the skin (Black 1873: 293). Edward Jarvis was even more stringent, recommending that a healthy person should bathe at least once a day (Jarvis 1845: 38). For a person suffering from illness, proper hygiene was essential to the restoration of health. Florence Nightingale wrote that the "noxious matter" produced by the ill person should be removed "from the system as rapidly as possible" in order to allow the pores of the body to breathe (Nightingale 1860: 94).

Nineteenth-century hygiene was not only a sanitary and medical concern but also a moral and distinctively bourgeois intervention. The "privatization of social bodily encounters," which led the middle-class to police their personal hygiene, conceal their bodily functions, and disguise their natural bodily odors, was a project deeply ingrained in the "development of capitalist modernity" (Hamilakis 2014: 20). While soap was mobilized abroad as a tool of colonialism, in the asylum it served the homologous purpose of civilizing what was savage in the lunatic. Although psychiatrists shared the Romantic belief in the healing qualities of the natural environment, theirs was a tightly controlled, sanitized, and domesticated version of "Nature." Similarly, when it came to health reform, the "healthy" body—one in tune with its "natural" state—was one that was disciplined, regulated, and stripped of its "noxious matter" and odors. The maintenance of this standard of hygiene posed a formidable challenge for asylum administrators. The work required to address the sanitary and medical needs of a single patient in the home was described by Florence Nightingale as occupying the full attention of the nurse, in addition to the family, physician, and servants. The task of the asylum administrator was to maintain the same standard of care for a population of hundreds, if not thousands of patients, in the face of water scarcity, rampant overcrowding, staff shortages, and a rapidly deteriorating building.

At the time of its establishment in 1833, the Worcester State Hospital became one of the first public institutions in the United States to feature indoor plumbing, a measure that administrators believed would ensure hygienic and comfortable living conditions for patients ("State hospital filings" 1837). The plumbing was installed by Thomas Pollard of Boston, who with Thomas Philpott had installed one of the first indoor toilets in a hotel, the Tremont House, in 1830 (ibid., Cocks 2001: 76, *A Description of Tremont House* 1830: 19). In 1836, Worcester added shower baths to its arsenal of hygienic facilities (Trustees' Notes 1836). Invented in the 1790s, the shower bath would have represented an "unusual luxury" for most of the population of Massachusetts at this time (Little 1972: 40); its presence distinguished the Worcester State Hospital as an institution at the forefront of hygienic technology, rivaled only by McLean Asylum in Boston, a private institution that catered to a wealthy clientele.

Despite the technological sophistication of the facilities, administrators faced an uphill battle to maintain the water supply and secure the proper disposal of sewage from the hospital. The water procured from a well dug at the time of the hospital's construction was quickly deemed "unfit" for the purpose (Annual Report 1841: 7). As a result, administrators decided to link the hospital to the natural springs on the property of Dr. F. W. Paine: a task that involved the laying of a lead pipe over 1.25 miles of land, across the properties of eight different landowners and over two public roads, using the labor of male patients to dig the trenches (Trustees' Notes 1833). Although the quality of the water procured in this fashion was satisfactory, the pipes supplying it often failed or were disturbed by the property owners, leading to a shortage of water in the asylum. Throughout the mid-nineteenth century, trustees frequently complained that "the water is not flowing" (Trustees' Notes 1864). Without water, attendants could not maintain proper hygiene in the hospital, nor could sewage be properly purged from the building. At least one outbreak of sickness among patients was attributed to the failure of the aqueduct.

While the water supply of the second hospital was more reliable, it came with its own set of problems. The source of the water was the nearby Bell Pond; originally a swamp, the pond became dry and clogged with decomposing vegetable matter in the summer, making the water in the hospital "offensive to sight and smell" and "draw[ing] complaint from the inmates" (Annual Report 1881: 17). After two decades of malodorous water, administrators managed to secure a connection to the city's supply. When that source failed for two days in the fall of 1906, leaving the entire institution of over a thousand patients without water, administrators recognized the need to maintain their own provision in case of such emergencies (Annual Report 1906: 8). The wells that were dug on the hospital property for this purpose were later determined to be located precariously near to the asylum's sewage disposal beds, leading to possible contamination (Annual Report 1910: 17). Administrators' quest for supplementary water sources continued for years. Travelers passing over the highway in front of the hospital in the 1910s and 1920s would have met with the sight of crews of "disturbed" patients (figure 4.1), overseen by attendants, digging ditches along the perimeter of the property for the aqueduct that would connect the hospital to the adjacent Lake Quinsigamond (figure 4.2) (Annual Report 1920: 21).

As the patient population of the second hospital burgeoned past the capacity of its plumbing system, sewage became an unpleasant and hazardous issue. Administrators had pondered the quandary of how to dispose of the accumulated waste of hundreds of patients and staff since the 1850s. The design of the second hospital was intended to obviate this problem by disposing of sewage beneath its fields, thereby fertilizing crops "without creating nuisance from odors" (Annual Report 1879: 17). Waste was routed from the asylum

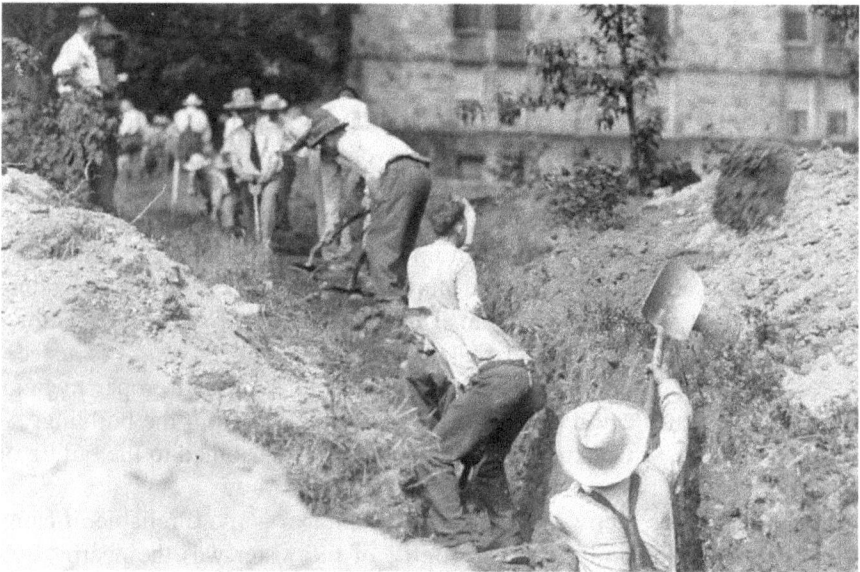

Figure 4.1   Patients Digging Ditches at the Second Worcester State Hospital in the Early Twentieth Century. The hospital depended upon these laborers, recruited from the ranks of the more tractable patients, to carry out projects such as the rerouting of the hospital aqueduct. *Source*: Courtesy of the Worcester Historical Museum.

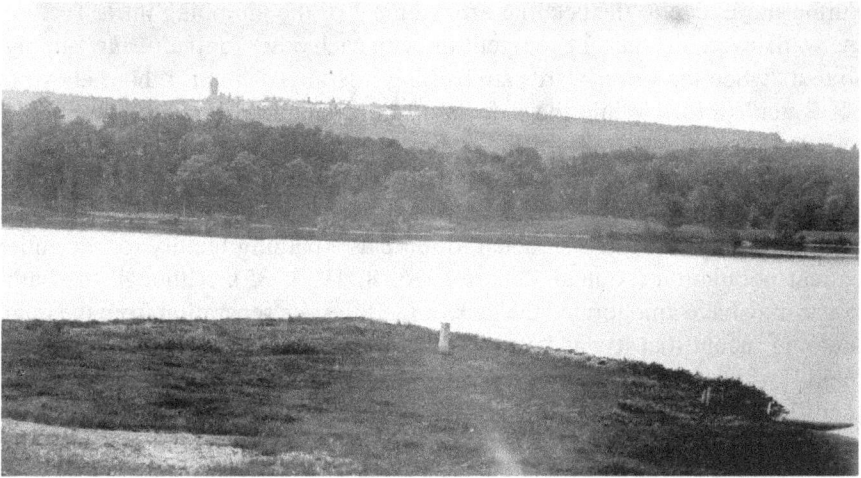

Figure 4.2   View of the Second Worcester State Hospital from across Lake Quinsigamond (in the Neighboring Town of Shrewsbury), Which Would Supply the Hospital with Water after Its Previous Source Was Deemed Inadequate. *Source*: Courtesy of the Worcester Historical Museum.

via three 12-inch cement pipes, corresponding to the central administrative building and its two wings, with access ports at regular intervals to allow the sewage to seep into the ground (ibid.: 16). However, the overburdening of this system and consequent overflow of raw sewage soon drew complaints from neighboring farmers and travelers on the highway that passed in front of the asylum (Annual Report 1914: 7). In 1904, the State Board of Health called attention to the asylum's sewer beds, which it feared posed the risk of polluting Lake Quinsigamond (Annual Report 1904: 8). Hoping to resolve what was rapidly becoming a "menace to the health of the adjacent community," trustees negotiated an arrangement with the city of Worcester in 1891 whereby the hospital would be linked to the city's sewers in exchange for a portion of the hospital property, which was to be converted into a park for city residents (Annual Report 1891). While the park quickly materialized, the city delayed fulfilling its part of the bargain for more than a quarter century, finally completing the link to the sewers in 1917 (Annual Report 1917).

The plumbing in the asylum building posed an additional challenge. The fixtures installed at the time of the second hospital's construction in 1877 were found to be obsolete by 1893, creating conditions that were "offensive" and a "menace to sanitary conditions" (Annual Report 1893: 6). Water closets and bathrooms were inconveniently located, "out of repair," and "hard to keep clean" (Annual Report 1892: 18). Bathing facilities were woefully inadequate, forcing groups of 40 to 60 patients to share a single tub.

Furthermore, due to the peculiar arrangement of the plumbing infrastructure, the wards were in constant competition with each other for their water supply, so that "when the lower wards are bathing it is impossible for those above to get water" (ibid.). While the defects of the system were easily identifiable, the cost of repair—$1000 for the central wards alone—posed a challenge to a hospital making do with a restrictive state budget. Complaints about the "antiquated conveniences" of the hospital persisted until the 1930s, when a central bathhouse was constructed to serve as a bathing facility for the entire patient population (Annual Report 1916: 8, 1933: 35). Although the bathhouse may have ameliorated the lack of facilities, its separation from the main building meant that it was "necessary to take patients out of doors to bathe them," which administrators described as "a decided hardship at any time, [and] in winter a positive cruelty" (ibid.).

THE ROLE OF ATTENDANTS

The limitations of institutional plumbing systems, poorly planned and almost immediately outdated, might have contributed to the fact that Clifford Beers often went weeks without a bath while housed in the violent ward of a Connecticut asylum. Beers, however, attributed it to the laziness of the attendants, who performed the bare minimum of the work that was needed to keep their charges alive and healthy (Beers 1913: 73). Elizabeth Packard also claimed that the personal hygiene of patients in the violent ward was badly neglected by their attendants. While confined to that ward, she made it her mission to bathe and groom her fellow patients, with remarkable results. "When the Doctor visited the ward that morning," she wrote, "I cannot forget the look of surprise he cast upon the row of clean faces and combed hair" (Packard 1873: 139). Turning the same meticulous attention to the ward itself, Packard reported proudly that "[o]urs [became] the neatest, best kept ward in the whole house; even the odor of which could not be surpassed in purity" (ibid.: 141). Beers's and Packard's accounts suggest that the asylum's human infrastructure—the corps of attendants and nurses who were charged with the care and treatment of patients—was as important to maintaining proper hygiene as the network of pipes and drains. However, like the hospital's plumbing systems, the staff often failed to meet the rigorous standards laid down by the administration.

Attendants occupied the frontlines in the battle against dirt and odor in the asylum, but were largely denied the respect and recompense that their position deserved. The occupation of asylum attendant was not a desirable one. Attendants were tasked with the discipline and management of psychotic patients and risked daily challenges to their health and well-being.

They worked 14-hour days, six days a week, and were poorly paid. Prior to the last decades of the nineteenth century, they were also almost universally untrained, arriving to the job with little understanding of insanity or its treatment. The low ratio of attendants to patients, present in almost every asylum in the country, increased this burden (Annual Report 1904: 12). Given these factors, it is unsurprising that attendants were not highly invested in their jobs and often remained for just as long as it took to find a better position (Annual Report 1866: 77, 1882: 18). Yet administrators placed an incredible amount of responsibility on attendants, expecting them to "devote their whole time and attention to patients," acting in the capacity of "friend," "adviser," "protector," and an exemplar to the insane in their "temper, manners, cheerfulness, activity, neatness, and order" (Conolly 1847: 110)—in addition to keeping their charges fed, clothed, and bathed, maintaining the cleanliness of the wards, administering medicine and other treatments, and supervising indoor and outdoor activities and labor.

Administrators lay much of the blame for the dysfunction of the asylum on the failure of attendants to meet these standards, attributing the abuse of patients to their attendants' inferior "moral and intellectual calibre" (Ray 1852: 52; Allen 1880: 6). It cannot be denied that some attendants were physically abusive toward patients, such violence was endemic to the institution and is described in virtually every patient account. However, these actions cannot be dissociated from the institutional system in which they were embedded. The role of systemic factors—such as staff shortages, low pay rates, lack of oversight and training, not to mention lack of effective treatments for violently insane patients—in enabling or encouraging certain behaviors in attendants was largely overlooked by administrators. Instead, they chose to target the individuals themselves, or more specifically, their ethnic and religious backgrounds.

At the time that the Worcester State Hospital was established, the pool of recruits from which the asylum drew its attendants was largely native-born. However, the growth of state hospitals—which generated a continuously growing demand for attendants—coupled with the rise of immigration into the United States meant that these positions were increasingly filled by immigrants. By the 1870s, psychiatrists had begun to complain about the changing demographic profile of attendants and its perceived effects on asylum administration. According to Isaac Ray,

> the character of attendants has been deteriorating . . . When I first went into this department of the healing art, the idea of having any other than our own people would have been most repulsive. Now, in most of our institutions, we find among the attendants different nationalities mixed up with our people. (Ray 1871)

Although Ellen Collins, a member of the New York County Committee of the State Board of Charities, shared some of this disdain toward the new class of attendants, she also expressed a degree of empathy with the challenges that they faced. In an 1874 letter, she challenged Pliny Earle's assertion that a postal department for the patients of asylums was unnecessary and would quickly become congested with the rambling letters of insane patients lodging false complaints against the institution. She proceeded to write:

> But would this apply to an Asylum like ours [Blackwell's Island] where 1400 women are crowded together, some of them in halls occupied by 75 to 90 patients under the care of two attendants, of whom a large part are Irish Roman Catholics, ignorant & liable to give practical expression to the impatience & irritability that spring from being desperately overworked & poorly paid? Do you not feel that the patients may some times have good ground for complaint? (Collins 1874)

Neither a physician nor an asylum administrator, Collins nonetheless possessed a degree of insight into the defects of the institution that those working on the inside of the asylum were often unable to achieve. To them, patients' complaints about the asylum were almost always dismissed as symptoms of their illness; any legitimate complaints could be conveniently assigned to the attendants themselves, rather than to their working conditions. As one trustee stated in the course of the 1902 nurses' strike, such grievances "are found to originate in the unbalanced minds of the unfortunate inmates or the revengeful dispositions of discharged employees" (*Worcester Sunday Herald* 1902).

Gerald Grob has described how the changing demographic profile of patients in the asylum affected how they were viewed and treated by their predominantly white, male, middle-class psychiatrists, leading to the undermining of moral treatment, which relied on a personal connection between individuals of shared social backgrounds and values (Grob 1966). Even Samuel B. Woodward, an icon of therapeutic optimism who was said to visit each of his two hundred patients daily, stated toward the end of his tenure at Worcester that "we are not so successful in our treatment of [the Irish] as with the native population of New England," and that it was "difficult to obtain their confidence" (Annual Report 1847: 33)—a word that specified the covenant of trust between psychiatrist and patient that formed the basis for moral treatment (Tomes 1984). This same dynamic shaped the interaction between psychiatrists and attendants, who served as the primary mediators between psychiatrists and patients and played the largest role in the everyday implementation of moral treatment. The asylum represented an agent of white, native-born, bourgeois morality; the efficacy of this model was therefore undermined by the presence of "outsiders" who represented alternative backgrounds and worldviews (Scull 1979: 183). The Irish were believed to be a separate race, different and distinctly inferior from their native-born counterparts. As patients, they were viewed as uncontrollable, resistant to treatment, and more likely to become incurably insane (Grob 1966: 139). As attendants, they were similarly uncontrollable, lazy, and therefore made poor emissaries for the moral lessons that administrators hoped they would impart to patients. Some historians have suggested that the proximity in socioeconomic position between patients and attendants contributed to attendants' abuse. Attendants who were "clinging tenaciously to the social ladder only a rung above many of the patients" were more likely to view patients with hostility as inferiors who were undeserving of the seemingly indulgent treatment that attendants were expected to lavish on them (Morrissey et al. 1980: 139). By keeping patients in their place, attendants policed the social hierarchies that sustained them on that slightly higher rung.

Unlike most state hospital patients, Clifford Beers and Elizabeth Packard came from educated, middle-class backgrounds (Beers had graduated from Yale; Packard's father and husband were ministers). This might help to explain why both chose to target attendants for the neglect of patients' hygiene. Notably, Packard identified one of the offending attendants in the violent ward as Irish, with a "unrefined and coarse nature" that contrasted with the "refined instincts" of the native-born attendant who had tended to Packard in the "better" ward (Packard 1873: 234–236). Elizabeth R. Hill, who had worked as a schoolteacher for almost twenty years, was similarly critical of the character of the attendants at the Worcester State Hospital, calling them "feeble-minded" (Hill 1881: 34).

This is not to say that such accounts were inaccurate; rather, that their views of the cleanliness (or lack thereof) of the asylum were refracted through their particular set of cultural values, which linked the domains of hygiene and health with morality and good character. Accordingly, the odor of the asylum was not simply an odor; it was "matter out of place," an affront to their personal worldviews and to the intended purpose of the asylum (Douglas 1966). Packard's effort to bathe her fellow patients not only served to remove dirt and odor but also represented a form of "personal redemption from the state of nature," which restored these patients to a "civilized state" (Bauman 1993: 24). The asylum was a bourgeois institution; as a member of bourgeois society herself, Packard's critique does not extend to the ideology or objectives of the asylum. Rather, she laments the fact that the asylum's failure to uphold its stated mission forced *her,* an individual, to shoulder the work of the institution in reclaiming the insane as members of civilized society. Hill rendered a similar assessment of the Worcester State Hospital, stating that it "ought to have capable physicians and nurses," instead of the "simple-minded" staff she had encountered during her commitment (Hill 1881: 20).

HYDROTHERAPY

In addition to its application in hygiene, water at asylums functioned as a therapeutic instrument that was thought to act directly on the mind and body. The notion of the healing powers of water has a long genealogy, dating back to the use of healing baths and springs in classical times. In 1584, Reginald Scot wrote that water, "both standing and running," contained "forces" that acted on the body in a way similar to certain medicines (Scot 1584: 165). Baths were espoused specifically for the treatment of "lunacy" as early as the seventeenth century (Cheyne 1642). Dutch physician Herman Boerhaave, writing in 1724, stated that the best treatment for madness was to "throw the Patient unwarily into the Sea, and keep him under Water as long as he can possibly bear without being quite stifled" (Boerhaave 1724: 303). Both Pinel and Esquirol espoused the use of baths as part of the earliest iterations of moral treatment.

By the nineteenth century, the ancient "water cure" had been appropriated by biomedicine, which linked the sensory experience of submersion to the achievement of certain mental states. In an article in the *American Journal of Insanity,* Ales Hrdlička wrote that the therapeutic "effects of water [were] produced chiefly through the physiological action of heat and cold upon the peripheral nervous system" (Hrdlička 1899: 444). The benefits of water were widely espoused by physicians and health reformers outside of asylums, such as Dr. M. G. Kellogg (Kellogg 1874: 9), who advocated the use of baths to regulate circulation, as well as temperance activists who believed that *"pure water* is the only physiological drink" (Stolz 1872: 49). Baths and springs were widely utilized by upper- and middle-class people seeking a particular combination of healthfulness, pleasure, and class distinction. Writing in the hospital's annual report in 1844, Woodward wrote that baths were the most extensively used "remedy" in the asylum (Annual Report 1844: 82). For this purpose, each of the galleries of the asylum was fitted with bathtubs and six shower baths. Warm baths and hot and cold packs were used to treat both acute mania and chronic insanity (figure 4.3). The second Worcester State Hospital featured a hydrotherapy department, with its own dedicated building constructed in 1910. By 1923, the department featured "thirteen continuous bath tubs," which were "in operation 24 hours a day" (Annual Report 1923: 7).

While psychiatrists insisted that hydrotherapy was applied exclusively as a therapeutic measure, multiple sources indicate its use as punishment, restraint, and means of control (Golden 1982: 122; Cherry 1989: 155). In the early nineteenth century, Benjamin Rush advocated the use of the shower bath as a means of disciplining recalcitrant patients (Rush 1872: 179). However, by the time the first state hospitals were established, most psychiatrists were

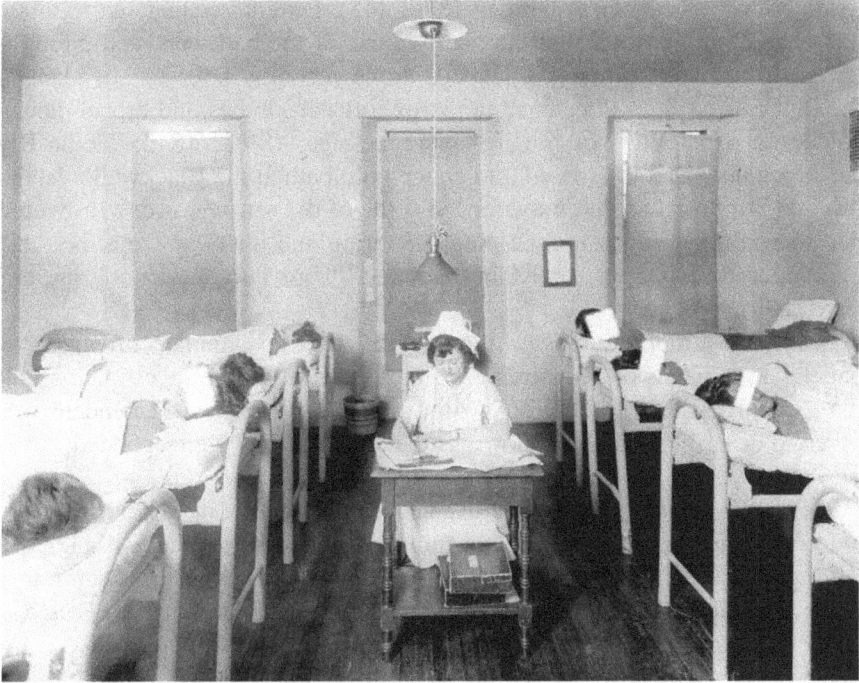

Figure 4.3   Patients undergoing Hydrotherapy at the Second Worcester State Hospital (Early Twentieth Century). Such treatments included the swaddling of patients in hot or cold towels for extended periods of time. *Source*: Courtesy of the Worcester Historical Museum.

at least nominally opposed to the use of baths as punishment, even as they acknowledged that baths *could* be weaponized against the inmates of institutions. Dorothea Dix endorsed the use of the shower bath as a "very effectual means of procuring submission to proper rules and regulations" in prisons, but made no such recommendation for asylums (Gollaher 1995: 211). Writing to Horace Mann in 1845, Woodward wrote that "[w]hipping is a cruel and degrading punishment, but the shower bath as practiced in Prison Discipline is often dangerous to life and should be strictly forbidden" (Woodward 1845). In an undated document in his personal papers, Woodward acknowledged that the cold bath was effective "if agreeable to the feelings of the patients, but like the circular swing it is too frequently considered as a punishment. The patient dreads its application and is frightened when it is applied. In such cases it is injurious rather than beneficial" (Woodward n.d.).

This advice was not always followed, according to a group of British psychiatrists who charged their American counterparts with using baths to punish patients in an 1876 editorial published in the London *Lancet* ("The treatment of insanity in America" 1876: 445). Patient accounts corroborate this charge and indicate that the punitive use of the bath persisted throughout the nineteenth century. Elizabeth Stone recounts how an attendant at the McLean Asylum threatened to "strip" off her clothes and drench her in cold water if she did not "control [her] feelings" (Stone 1842). Nellie Bly described how she was forced into an ice-cold bath at the Blackwell's Island Asylum, writing that she "experienced some of the sensations of a drowning person as they dragged me, gasping, shivering and quaking, from the tub." She added that as a result of this treatment, "[f]or once I did look insane" (Bly 1887).

Several testimonies indicate the use of water to simulate drowning in patients as a means of disciplining them. As part of a state investigation into the Central Kentucky Lunatic Asylum in the 1880s, its superintendent was asked to describe a practice known as the "towel bath." He responded:

The towel bath is nothing more than confining the hands of the patient and the feet to keep them from kicking or striking the patients or patients assisting. A towel of dipped in water and laid over the face. It produces a feeling of suffocation, and the patient soon gives up and becomes tractable. That remedy is used in every institution in the United States. (Hurd 1883: 506–507)

Dr. Henry Hurd, who reported on the investigation for the *American Journal of Insanity,* claimed that "my object in writing this brief note is to protest against these statements," which "do not represent the views and practices of the AMSAII." However, at least one account supports the superintendent's claim that the "towel bath"—or similar practices—was widely used in American asylums. Moses Swan reports being the victim of such a "remedy" as an inmate of the Troy Lunatic Asylum in the 1870s:

I was there ordered into a bath tub of cold water, compelled to sit down, compelled to lie down, bound as I was hand and foot, and chilled through and through; my feet were pressed hard against the foot of the bath tub and my shoulders against the raised bottom of the tub. The water not being of sufficient depth over the raised part of the bottom to cover my head or keep it under water, the attendant took an old tin wash dish, and dipping the water from between my legs poured the dirty water into my mouth and down my throat, keeping my mouth pried open all the while. I begged for my life; I cried for mercy; they would not desist, but again and again filled the dish and poured it down my throat. I was almost strangled, but not yet content, they both grabbed my legs and raised them from the bottom of the tub, thereby drawing my head and shoulders into the deeper water. Then the attendant, by the aid of Scott, held my head under water until I was almost strangled. Whenever I was almost gone they would raise it a moment for me to revive, and then jam it down again under the water. (Swan 1874: 5)

While most psychiatrists may not have openly endorsed the use of water in this way, several describe its use to shock and intimidate patients into submission. Frederic Skey described a phenomenon common to hysteric wards whereby the "fits" exhibited by one patient acted like a contagion, leading to the expression of similar symptoms in other patients simultaneously. His solution was to throw cold water on one of the agitated patients, which inevitably caused the cessation of the fit in the others (Skey 1867: 60). Pliny Earle described the use of a similar "treatment" in the case of a hysterical patient:

> A lady who, for many months, had been subject to the almost daily recurrence of a species of fits, in which she was prostrated and violently convulsed was admitted into a hospital. The physician in her presence directed her nurse to keep a pail of water standing in her room, and the moment the fit seized her, to dash it upon her. From that hour the fits never returned. This was hydropathy [*sic*] in its perfection. (Earle 1858)

These practices demonstrate the use of "hydrotherapy" in precisely the way that Woodward warned was "injurious" to the patient: as a fear tactic, employed to secure control. The weaponization of hydrotherapy in asylums represented a grotesque mirror image of the elite use of baths. In both cases, the bath served as a "tool of social division" (Bauman 1993: 25), marking one class of people as inferior, deviant, and deserving of the cleansing effects of the bath to purge them of their filth and savagery, and the other as superior, physically and morally pure, and worthy of the effects of the bath as a pleasurable sensuous experience.

Even as they repudiated the punitive function of the bath, psychiatrists acknowledged that it served as a form of control when they described it as a substitute for other forms of restraint. In 1906, the administrators of the Worcester State Hospital reported that "in place of drugs and mechanical restraint," they now used "the hot pack and prolonged bath to allay excitement and sleeplessness" (Annual Report 1906: 12). The discourse surrounding hydrotherapy suggests the complicated and overlapping position it occupied between treatment and restraint. This muddy boundary speaks to the ambiguous nature of the asylum itself. Was the function of the asylum to cure or to control? And was there a difference? To nineteenth-century psychiatrists, a "cured" patient was one who acted normally, that is, in accordance with the standards of asylum discipline and social norms, whether or not his internal symptoms (e.g., negative emotions, hallucinations, compulsive thoughts) had resolved. This result could be achieved by "curing" the patient of his illness, or by intimidating, deceiving, beating, drowning, or medicating the patient into submission. Could a patient who no longer resisted attendants' demands due to the fear of being submerged in an ice-cold bath be considered "improved?" When it came to determining the status of patients' disease, nineteenth-century psychiatrists relied largely on the externalized manifestations of mental illness rather than on its interior experience, giving primacy to their own senses over the patients. It was not until the advent of psychoanalysis that psychiatrists foregrounded the interiority of mental illness.

In the nineteenth century, however, many psychiatrists were cognizant of the inherent limitations of their discipline in identifying and targeting the root causes of insanity. Even those treatments that were widely touted as effective were largely indistinguishable from the remedies of their predecessors. In his annual report of 1844, Isaac Ray wrote that "he would be a bold man who should venture to say that Pinel and Esquirol, whose medical treatment was confined chiefly to baths and simple bitter drinks, were less successful in their cure of mental diseases than those numerous practitioners who have exhausted upon them all the resources of the healing art" (Earle 1887: 529). Like music and narcotic medicines, the primary utility of hydrotherapy was to tranquilize the patient, temporarily masking symptoms while leaving the underlying pathology unchanged. Partly for this reason, hydrotherapy was largely abandoned following the emergence of the first psychoactive medicines, which—although they did not cure mental illness—eliminated symptoms with unprecedented and unambiguous efficacy. Although critics of psychiatry would claim that these medicines represented yet another manifestation of social control, they had the distinct effect of dissociating that function from the asylum. Unlike moral treatment, which depended on the immersive, isolated, and stationary institutional environment, the new pharmacological therapeutics was mobile, untethered to any particular site.

THE SMELL OF THE INSANE

In the early modern era, popular belief attributed distinctive, unpleasant odors to certain deviant individuals. The "sickening smell" exuded by witches was cited as an olfactory signifier of their diabolical associations, as though their bodies had literally putrefied as a result of their consort with the devil (Barstow 1994: xiv). As skepticism toward the existence of witchcraft spread, however, and the medico-scientific model began to exert its claim over phenomena that had previously been attributed to the supernatural, beliefs surrounding malodorous "witches" were reinterpreted. In 1718, Francis Hutchinson wrote that the "Rank Unsavoury Smell" exuded by some old women as a result of "Poverty, and old Age, and bad Diet, and want of convenient Linnen," provoked an "Antipathy" in their neighbors that might subconsciously plant the seed for witchcraft accusations (Hutchinson 1718: 3). Thus, it was the odor—as it was refracted through neighbors' vindictive and paranoid minds—that put the (perception of) evil into the woman, rather than the evil that produced the odor.

In the nineteenth century, disease came to replace the devil as the attributed cause for the unpleasant smells of the body. Insanity was among the ailments that were said to be "indicated by the odour of the patient's excretions" (Johnson 1856: 102). Etienne Esquirol described the smell of the insane as "a penetrating odor, impregnating both the clothing and furniture, and which nothing can remove" (Esquirol 1845: 27). In 1844, Samuel B. Woodward noted that the perspiration of certain patients at the Worcester State Hospital "emits an odor quite peculiar and very offensive, [rendering] cleanliness and ventilation important" (Annual Report 1844: 86). Similarly, distinctive and repugnant smells were attributed to the sufferers of neurasthenia and to masturbators (Van Deusen 1869: 12). The linkage of odors to certain diseases meant that the olfactory was claimed as a sensory domain that could be marshaled in the pursuit of medical knowledge. With this "translation of olfactory vigilance into scientific language," the physician's nose was enlisted alongside his eyes and ears as an instrument in the rituals of diagnosis (Corbin 1986: 14). Yet because the traditional hierarchy by which the senses were ordered was maintained, the olfactory—as one of the "lower" sensory orders—never occupied the same status or level of importance that was accorded to vision or hearing.

The insane were not the only class of individuals to whom unpleasant odors were attributed on account of their supposedly aberrant biologies. The characteristic traits of the insane overlapped with other categories of difference, tapping into intersecting concerns with public health, social organization, and the containment of the Other. One of these categories was race. Woodward noted the existence of an "odor given off by diseased persons or those of dirty habits, and particularly by blacks," which "indicates the presence of those poisonous matters, which are ever obnoxious to health" (Woodward 1839). This statement fetters difference to disease, implicating a common racist belief within the biomedical paradigm, and thereby medicalizes blackness as biologically distinct and pathologically deviant (Thomas 1991). Echoing Woodward's statements regarding the "offensive" perspiration of the insane, physician William H. Holcombe wrote that "[t] he black skin of the negro exhales, especially when heated, a very offensive perspiration" (Smith 2006: 45–46). By mobilizing similar rhetoric to describe insanity and blackness, physicians legitimized the status of both as categories of biological alterity. The implication was that blacks were not simply of a different race but a distinctly inferior one; just as insanity represented a deviation from sanity, blackness represented a deviation from whiteness.

There were many parallels between how blacks and the insane were conceptualized and treated, as members of a deviant class that were believed to require control and containment by social and physical restraints (Gilman 1985: 148). Many of the characteristics that were used to define blackness and insanity, respectively, had to do with the ways in which these "deviant" individuals sensed, or were sensed by, others. Whites used their senses to "detect" blackness in the same way that physicians used their senses to diagnose insanity, building off the assumption that these categories were "sensorily distinctive" (Smith 2006: 12); that is, blacks and lunatics looked, sounded, and smelled differently from their "normal" counterparts. Additionally, the sensoria of blacks and lunatics were thought to function differently. A common belief among white people was that black people were less sensitive than they were to pain. Similarly, prior to the rise of moral treatment, the insane were thought to be insensible to pain, heat, and cold (Wynter 2010: 43). In both cases, notions of the Other's altered sensibility served to justify how they were treated. A black person who could not feel pain could be subjected to hard labor and corporal punishment (Smith 2006: 46). Likewise, a lunatic who could not feel pain or cold could be chained in an unheated and unfurnished cell.

In the nineteenth century, beliefs surrounding the sensibility of the insane reversed. Under the paradigm of moral treatment, lunatics were believed to be *more* sensitive to sensory stimuli than the sane, a fact which was used to legitimize physicians' control over every aspect of their environment. In the same way that "justifications for the continuation of bondage" were "embedded in sensory representations of blackness," the discourse surrounding the senses and sensibility of the insane were deeply implicated in the ideology of confinement (Smith 2006). Blacks and the insane were both set aside as classes that were incapable of independence, a belief that justified their subjection to paternalistic regimes of discipline (Reiss 2008: 53). Unlike blackness, however, insanity was—at least for a brief period—believed to be curable. The total institution held out the promise that deviant individuals could be "corrected," shorn of their aberrant qualities, and refashioned into normative, productive citizens. The immutability of race presented a provocation to this institutional ideology. Early European discourses on race suggested that the skin color of blacks might lighten once they were assimilated to white lifeways (Smith 2006). Long after this theory was abandoned, blacks continued to be punished for their "failure" to become white, either physically or culturally. Though deliberately set apart from society, the asylum did not provide a reprieve from society's racism; on the contrary, as the designated enforcer of "bourgeois morality" and its correspondent philosophies of difference

(Foucault 1977), it served to fortify racial hierarchies. Most asylums in the South disallowed black patients altogether, while northern asylums practiced varying degrees of segregation. In June of 1833—when the Worcester State Hospital had been open for less than six months—its trustees noted the need for separate "arrangements for the Africans, who ought not to mingle with the other female patients" (Trustees' Notes 1833). In July, they reported that "the Commissioners for erecting the buildings have caused six rooms to be prepared in one of the buildings for the confinement of the worst class of female patients and the few black women." In October 1833, trustee W. B. Calhoun wrote that "the separation of the Africans from the rest of the inmates answers fully the purpose intended, and they are very comfortably lodged" (ibid.). This "purpose" undoubtedly was to ensure the comfort of white patients and staff, rather than that of the black patients.

Black patients were not the only ones set apart in the Worcester State Hospital. The Irish were also separated into their own wards, a practice that was endorsed by Dorothea Dix, who further suggested that Irish patients be removed from the asylum entirely to provide space for "our citizens" (Gollaher 1995: 344). Irish patients were blamed for their own insanity— which Woodward attributed to "want of forethought in them to save earnings for a day of sickness, indulgence in stimulating drinks, and strong love for their native land" (Annual Report 1847: 33)—and disdained by administrators for their failure to contribute to the cost of their treatment at the asylum (Annual Report 1849: 37). Not coincidentally, the Irish—in addition to other groups, such as Italians and Jews—were also targeted by middle-class hygienic reformers who viewed them as dirty and disease-ridden. Just as Irish lunatics were blamed for their own insanity, the immigrant inhabitants of urban slums were blamed for their own uncleanliness and disease. As "odor intolerance became a defining feature of social status for the middle classes," lack of hygiene and its correspondent odors became indexes of inferiority both inside and outside of the asylum (Hamilakis 2014: 20). In its function as a machine of sanitization, the asylum served the project of bourgeois modernity in defining and shaping reality through its olfactory dimensions. The "smell of the insane" served as a metonym for the broader concept of the smell of deviance, an olfactory signifier that was as visceral and imbued with social meaning as the bygone scent of the witch.

According to Mark M. Smith, black people challenged the idea of a "black odor" by stating that if they smelled differently from whites, it was not due to their biological makeup, but to the sweat-inducing physical labor, they were forced to endure as slaves and free people (ibid.). Their odor, they claimed, was the product of racism, not race. The filth and disease attributed to immigrants were the products of their marginalization in crowded and poorly designed tenement buildings. Likewise, it seems probable that the distinctive "smell of the insane" was in many cases caused not by insanity, but by institutionalization. Perhaps the most offensive smells associated with patients were attributable to the asylum's faulty ventilation and plumbing systems and the failure to maintain a decent standard of hygiene. These odors were not intrinsic to insanity, but rather were produced by the particular architectural and administrative configurations of the asylum, whereby hundreds—and ultimately thousands—of patients were crowded into outmoded facilities that had been designed to hold only a fraction of that number. It is particularly telling that physicians looked instinctively to individual deviance—rather than to the system—for an explanation for the characteristic odor of the insane. This same logic was widely mobilized in ideologies of race, gender, class, and nativity throughout the nineteenth century, and played a major role in fueling the growth of the institution as bourgeois society's default solution for the pathologies of the individual.

Equally important to explaining the "smell of the insane" is the culture-bound expectation that bodies should *not* smell. Although the human sense of smell is universal, the value to which different smells are assigned, and the belief that they should or should not exist, are historically specific. The emergence of the asylum coincided with the development of a particular set of "sensorial hierarchies," which "merged with colonial practices of appropriation, slavery, and subjugation, as well as practices having to do with sanitisation and the 'civilizing' of the collective body at 'home'" (Hamilakis 2014: 34). To ascribe a certain smell to the insane was not simply to describe or diagnose them, but to locate them within a sensorial hierarchy that cast the malodorous as inferior and demanded that "smells were to be disciplined" (Bauman 1993: 25–26). While the vagaries of architectural and administrative practice can help us to understand why the asylum failed, a deeper understanding of the asylum demands that we articulate the genealogies and social meaning embedded in the objectives it was tasked to meet.

CONCLUSION

Dorothea Lynde Dix lived long enough to see much of the promise of her reforms fall through (Gollaher 1995). The vivid descriptions of the filth and odor of the strong rooms where the violently insane were confined in nineteenth-century asylums bear an uncomfortable resemblance to the conditions described by Dix and other mental health reformers who visited lunatics living in makeshift accommodations across the state prior to the establishment of asylums (Deutsch 1946: 183). For these patients, the asylum may not have represented much of an improvement over their previous condition. This fact was acknowledged in a report of the House of

Commons Select Committee assigned to investigate conditions in English asylums, which noted "how closely the complaints and aims of the reformers, in the days when there were few county or borough asylums, resemble our own. It is in respect to the very evils these . . . institutions were designed to remedy that they are themselves conspicuously defective" (Scull 1979: 219).

Out of all the promises made by the asylum, the guarantee of a clean, habitable living space occupied the foundation of the pyramid in its particular hierarchy of needs. The asylum was one of many total institutions: technologies of modernity that were aimed at processing the rougher orders of society into more refined ones. Accordingly, the asylum was stationed at the vanguard of modernity's "war on smells," aimed not only at sanitizing the individual lunatic, but at purging humanity of its last "vestige of animality" (Bauman 1993: 25). The futility of trying to extract foul odors from the air, of scrubbing clean the "intangible atmosphere," of pumping air and water through degraded infrastructure, of cleansing bodies that continuously exuded "noxious" waste and smeared themselves with excrement—all came to represent the Sisyphean nature of the task faced by asylum administrators. The failure of hygiene and sanitation was both a literal example and ideological statement of the broader futility of the asylum, and directly challenged the very premise of moral treatment. What good were scenic vistas and pleasant music when the insane were confined to filthy, foul-smelling cells? How could psychiatrists claim the asylum as a humane, scientific solution to the problem of insanity when it failed to provide accommodations that were better than the "cages, closets, cellars, stalls, [and] pens" decried by Dix?

In their ongoing efforts to bring the olfactory domain of the asylum into alignment with its intended sensorial regime, administrators made several crucial mistakes of attribution. Their focus on individual deviance, as embodied in the diseased physiology of patients and the compromised "moral and intellectual calibre" of attendants, represented a stubborn refusal to assign the proper significance to structural issues in the physical and ideological framework of the asylum. This faulty logic is most clearly represented in continuing belief in the "smell of the insane," a concept that allowed psychiatrists to neatly circumscribe the issue of odor within the physical body of the lunatic, thus absolving the asylum of its fault in producing odors and its need to remedy the situation. Because "Otherness [is] defined partly by odour, especially when odours are embodied and emanate from the body of the other" (Hamilakis 2014: 18), the notion that certain individuals—whether insane, black, or immigrants—exuded certain signature, unpleasant smells was promulgated by the asylum and helped to contribute to the belief that the asylum's mission was inherently futile: not because of its own defects, but because of the immutable defectiveness of deviant individuals.

Thus, administrators' realization that asylums would never be the "uto-pias" they had imagined went hand in hand with the growing conviction that insanity was largely incurable. Both sentiments were products of the appar-ent failure of the asylum to deliver on its promise to cure insanity through the environment. Yet it is unclear how much this failure had to do with the inherent impossibility of the promises made, and how much it derived from the matrix of historical contingencies into which the asylum model was cast. How would the asylum have looked—or more precisely, smelled—if it had been properly furnished with funds and other resources, equipped with a well-paid and well-trained corps of attendants, and relieved of overcrowding? Is it possible for a system founded on the primacy of the institutional model to acknowledge its own role in producing dysfunction and harming patients? Psychiatrists agreed that an asylum that could not provide a clean, salutary environment was an asylum that could not cure; and an asylum that could not cure was nothing but a prison, a human warehouse. Yet they never had the opportunity—or the insight—to properly assess the inverse of that theory: that an asylum that could provide a proper environment was one that could substantially improve the lives of the mentally ill.

NOTE

1. These included the cottage plan, which was resisted for most of the nineteenth century before being reluctantly embraced in the early twentieth, and the Gheel model, which never gained traction in the United States.

Chapter 5

Dirty Bread, Forced Feeding, and Tea Parties

The Uses and Abuses of Food

Nineteenth-century psychiatrists assigned food—its production, nutritional content, and the behaviors surrounding its consumption—a major role in the program of moral treatment. In doing so, they drew upon an extensive legacy of ancient and early modern knowledge, which offered guidelines for achieving a healthy mind and body. Notably, these guidelines were not purely medical in nature, but made explicit connections between dietary health and moral values. In *The Anatomy of Melancholy* (1621), Robert Burton identified improper diet as a contributor to both physical and mental disorder, claiming that "gluttony"—one of the seven deadly sins—"kills more than the sword" (Burton 1621: 196). The link between food and morality would persist into nineteenth-century medicine. In his 1873 treatise *The Ten Laws of Health*, physician J. R. Black traced the entanglement of morals and food to the Bible, attributing mankind's discovery "that there are such things as good and evil" to the consumption of "forbidden fruits" (Black 1873: 86).

Although they were increasingly disinclined to explicitly invoke the Bible or God, nineteenth-century psychiatrists endorsed essentially the same rules as their early modern predecessors, which they reframed within a biomedical model predicated on "natural" ways of living. As Nature came to stand as a desacralized proxy for the divine within medicine, it assumed a God-like role in arbitrating the rules of the universe and doling out correspondent rewards and punishments. Individuals who obeyed the rules of Nature would be rewarded with good health, while violators were penalized with illness and infirmity. Woodward wrote that "transgressions of the laws of life," such as "eat[ing] excessively . . . will be followed by summary punishment, as surely as violations of the moral law" (Annual Report 1845: 61).

Although the religious genealogies underlying these discourses were largely mystified in the process of their appropriation by medical experts, certain rhetorical legacies were preserved. Physician John Harvey Kellogg called his rules for dietary hygiene "commandments" (similar to Black's "ten laws"), a term that carried the authority of the divine and foreclosed the possibility for alternative points of view. Kellogg's commandments mandated that meals be taken at the same time of day each day; that food be eaten neither too much nor too frequently; that vegetables should be preferred over meat; that "hot and stimulating drinks" be avoided, as they were "detrimental to health"; and fats and oils be eschewed entirely (Kellogg 1874: 10–17). Both the content of the "commandments" and their moral overtones were largely resonant with those endorsed by psychiatrists.

Insanity occupied a prominent place in the catalog of illnesses that could be precipitated by the violation of natural laws. Modern ways of living were thought to be "artificial," that is, discordant with the rules of nature. Psychiatrists believed that the high prevalence of mental diseases in the nineteenth century was a distinctively modern phenomenon. However, in conceptualizing this phenomenon, they drew upon long-established medical aphorisms. Centuries before insanity was described as a "disease of civilization," early modern physicians had implicated the violation of the laws of health—and specifically dietary laws—in the etiology of insanity. In 1642, English physician George Cheyne identified "*Mal-regimen* of Diet" as a primary cause of "True *Mania's* [sic], real *Lunacy, Madness,* and a disorder'd Brain" (Cheyne 1642). Similarly, Richard Burton—drawing on Fernelius—identified "diet [as] the mother of diseases," stating that "from this alone melancholy and frequent other maladies arise" (Burton 1621: 190).

In the context of an industrializing and colonialist society, food and its consumption were inevitably drawn into discourses of progress, culture, and evolution. Here, physicians faced a quandary. The type, preparation, and consumption of food were afforded key roles in defining civilization and distinguishing modern people from the lower orders of humanity. According to Black, "[t]he barbarian takes food and drink as prepared by nature," while "the man of culture as modified by art" (Black 1873: 84). These postures of gentility were essential to marking Westerners as culturally and intellectually superior, yet physicians believed that their departure from "natural" ways of living exerted pernicious effects on health. Because "barbarians" lived in a state of nature, they were spared the "diseases of civilization." On the other hand, the "sensualism" and "over-adequateness" exhibited by modern people represented a violation of natural laws (ibid.). Nature, in turn, responded by inscribing the stigmata of this violation onto the offenders' bodies. Physicians bemoaned the fact that while "savages" and American slaves enjoyed "excellent and beautiful teeth," refined young women were forced to use dentures (ibid.: 90). Digestive and sexual disorders, intemperance, and insanity were likewise counted among the afflictions that were imposed as punishment for artificiality and indulgence.

Despite their belief that civilization was to blame for much of the disease and debility suffered by modern people, physicians did not suggest that their patients revert to a state of savagery in order to preserve their health; rather, they recommended education in order to bring modern people back into alignment with the rules of nature while retaining the graces and comforts of society. According to physicians, the privileges of civilization came along with a particular set of temptations that the uneducated masses were poorly equipped to resist. Books such as Black's *Ten Laws* and Kellogg's *Hygienic Family Physician* were targeted at these masses, encouraging the assumption of an ascetic, "natural" diet in defiance of the abundance and artifice of modern society. A meal should consist "of as few articles as possible: bread, meat, one kind of vegetable. Temperance in diet, water for drink, and hard work for exercise will save and prolong life" (Culverwell 1848: 21). Moderation was the law of nature; extremes in either direction were unnatural and should be avoided. The fear of illness and infirmity served to discipline the readers of these texts into conformity with the authors' "commandments." The specter of insanity would have presented a particularly powerful incentive to obey the rules of nature. After all, the lunatic suffered not only from the loss of his reason but also from the stigma surrounding insanity: a stigma that was reinforced by physicians' assertion that lunatics were transgressors of natural laws.

THE LAW OF MODERATION

In explaining how diet led to insanity, psychiatrists targeted opposite ends of a social spectrum that was increasingly polarized. On the one hand, they claimed, insanity could be caused by "sensualism" and "overindulgence," as exhibited by the upper and middle classes; on the other, it could be caused by the privation and starvation that afflicted the poor. Starvation led to the "deterioration" of the body, which in turn sapped the brain of energy, causing "the manifestations of mind [to] fail [along] with the other functions" (Conolly 1847: 66). Once established, insanity could also work to deaden the appetite, leading to a vicious cycle of worsening mental health. Accordingly, a lack of adequate nutrition was viewed as both a contributor to and a symptom of insanity (Griesinger 1866: 331). The effects of starvation on the mind were so radical that in certain cases the provision of adequate food was thought to be sufficient to improve and even cure mental disease (ibid.).

The beliefs held by superintendents at state hospitals such as Worcester may have been influenced by the fact that many—if not most—of their patients belonged to the lower strata of society. Many "pauper lunatics" suffered at the time of their admission from some degree of malnutrition and other physical effects of poverty, which doubtlessly affected the expression of their symptoms. Accordingly, it is not surprising that superintendent Samuel B. Woodward believed that "insanity frequently seems to be produced by insufficient diet" (Annual Report 1843: 75). Yet even those physicians who worked at private institutions—such as Isaac Ray, the superintendent of the Butler Hospital in Rhode Island—corroborated this claim, despite the fact that the cases of insanity they treated were more likely to be attributed to overindulgence than to want.

The dangers posed to mental health by overindulgence stemmed from the overstimulation of the senses. Physicians believed that too great a focus on sensory pleasures in the form of "animal food" gave "undue ascendancy to the lowest propensities, leading to aberration and insanity" (Fowler 1856: 27–28). While the pauper insane often suffered from food scarcity, psychiatrists accused them of overindulgence in drink, a discursive gesture that conveniently shifted blame back onto the individual and away from structural inequalities. According to Black, intemperance was "the most influential of all exciting causes of insanity among the lower classes" (Black 1873: 132). Most American psychiatrists prohibited the recreational use of alcohol in asylums and were shocked to learn that abstinence was not enforced by their British counterparts. Visiting the Chesire Lunatic Asylum in 1860, Edward Jarvis reported to his wife that beer "being a very common drink here, it is given to patients who need to live well" (Jarvis 1860). The stance against alcohol taken by American psychiatrists can be attributed to their membership in the Protestant, native-born upper-middle class, which at the time was experiencing a swell of temperance enthusiasm that openly linked the use of alcohol with immorality, degeneration, and vice. Some psychiatrists, such as Pliny Earle, went a step further in also condemning the use of tea and coffee (Earle 1858).

In addition to alcohol, nineteenth-century American psychiatrists also identified certain types of food as contributors to insanity, a claim that derived partly from earlier Galenic models of medicine based on the existence of humors. According to humoral theory, physical and mental health were dependent upon the equilibrium of the various substances that composed the body. Excessive consumption of one variety of food could throw off this balance, leading to illness. Accordingly, Burton counseled the melancholic to avoid beef, "strong and hearty," which was productive of "gross melancholy blood" (Burton 1621: 190). While nineteenth-century physicians no longer believed in the existence of humors, they claimed that certain substances—including "alcohol, bad food, tobacco, tea, coffee, opium, henbane, hops, chloral," and "polluted air"—acted like poisons in the blood, and could produce insanity. Neurasthenia was said to be "a food disease," resulting from the "fermentat[ion]" of certain types of food in the alimentary canal, leading to paralysis and mental disorder; treatment involved the substitution of foods that would clear the digestive system properly (Holbrook 1878: 59).

Psychiatrists' beliefs surrounding the "proper" amount and quality of food, the evils of overindulgence and intemperance, and the dichotomous opposition of civilization and nature were inflected by their moral values. In presenting these beliefs as objective standards derived from Nature, they denied the possibility of legitimate alternatives. For example, while recognizing that individuals exhibited different tastes in food, psychiatrists believed that these differences were learned, not innate, representing deviations from the body's natural predilections. "Natural taste," wrote Black, "when left to itself, selects precisely the kind of food suitable for the body" (Black 1873: 112). Taste became corrupted when "dishes [were] made so palatable that the temptation to over-eat is almost irresistible" (ibid.). Similarly, Stolz wrote that "sense" was "wonderfully perverted by disobedience to its mandates," specifically the use of "artificial stimulants, acrid and narcotic substances . . . Pernicious habits lessen sensibility and destroy the natural relish for healthful food and drink" (Stolz 1872: 86). Such perversions were not only threatening to health but also to "moral and intellectual development" (ibid.).

The theory of violation provided the connecting link between immorality and mental pathology, enabling the inscription of social standards—such as the "laws" of moderation, intemperance, and productivity—into medical etiologies. These rules reflected the social backgrounds of medical practitioners who generally belonged to the upper-middle class and drew upon Calvinist and Quaker value systems that valued a hard-working, ascetic lifestyle. To members of this class, the unhealthy, intemperate, or insane person was guilty of a double offense: violation of the laws of nature as well as the laws of society. As a result of the entanglement of medical knowledge with moral concepts of sin and punishment, psychiatrists were primed to view their patients—and particularly those of the morally inferior lower classes—as offenders rather than victims. This, in turn, influenced whether psychiatrists viewed their patients as worthy or unworthy, curable or incurable.

Although upper- and middle-class patients were also seen as violators of social norms, psychiatrists were more likely to be more sympathetic toward these failings and even to see them as valuable. While lower-class patients' illnesses were attributed to their crudeness, ignorance, and laziness, neurotic symptoms in the upper classes were often seen as by-products of sensitivity, refinement, and intelligence—a belief that contributed to the "fashionable embrace of nervous disorders" among the latter (Scull 2009: 52). Not only were psychiatrists more accepting of the mental afflictions particular to their

class, they were more likely to suffer from them personally or know some-
one who did. In 1878 John D. Washburn, a trustee of the Worcester State
Hospital, suffered from a nervous breakdown that was attributed in the press
to the mental strain of his responsibilities as a politician and businessman, as
well as to "the care and anxiety incidental to the erection of the new hospital
for the insane" (Washburn Papers 1878). Ironically, his physician, fellow
trustee Thomas Gage, prescribed a trip to Havana—rather than a stay in the
new hospital—as treatment. Likewise Merrick Bemis, the superintendent of
Worcester State Hospital, sought treatment for his depressive moods not at
his own public institution, but at the private Pennsylvania Hospital for the
Insane (Tomes 1984: 279).

Social class thus played a major role in shaping the diagnosis and treatment of patients in the asylum. Disdain and pity on the part of the psychiatrist toward the patient were inimical to the process of confidence building
and mutual respect that was considered essential to moral treatment, and
contributed to psychiatrists' belief that the lower classes were less amenable
to—and less worthy of—treatment. Even Woodward, who was renowned
for his sympathy for his patients, suffered from this prejudice, particularly
toward Irish paupers.

TREATMENT: CONSUMPTION AND PRODUCTION

If insanity could be caused by "Mal-regimen of diet," it seemed logical
that treatment would necessitate the substitution of proper dietary habits.
Psychiatrists believed that even those patients whose insanity wasn't caused
directly by poor diet could benefit from the consumption of a certain quality
and quantity of food. In the first decades of the Worcester State Hospital,
administrators spoke proudly of their dietary, claiming that the wholesome
and appetizing meals served at the hospital would bolster the physical well-
being of their patients, which in turn would promote their return to sanity.
Woodward described the hospital diet as "[s]imple and substantial food,"
consisting of "meat [at least] once a day . . . . bread of the best quality,
vegetables in season, coffee in the morning and tea at night," and claimed
that the menu was "never the same two days in succession" (Annual Report
1840: 77).

Because both upper and lower classes of patients were guilty of transgress-
ing nature's laws, psychiatrists believed that the asylum dietary should be
aimed at equalizing both of them, aiming for a state of "natural" moderation.
Accordingly, John Conolly advised that "[d]iet should be for the insane pauper more liberal and nutritious than usually found in his cottage," and "for
the wealthier patient simpler and plainer than that usual at his own table"

(Conolly 1847: 70). W. A. F. Browne proposed a system based on the incentivizing of certain varieties of food and other "coveted luxuries" as rewards for labor, arguing that the preferential treatment of certain patients—at least in regards to diet—should be based on merit rather than status (Browne 1837: 197). Similarly, George Parkman suggested that the "quantity of food [should be] proportioned to activity," as an "inducement to employment" (Parkman 1817: 18). Because upper-class patients were less inclined to work than their lower-class counterparts, a meritocratic system would have mainly benefited the latter.

Woodward claimed that unlike British institutions, which maintained hierarchies of "5-6 classes [of patients], each with different food," at Worcester "we make little distinction in the ordinary diet, directing from time to time such as particular individuals may require" (Annual Report 1843: 70). These requirements were based on medical need, such as "convalescents from mania" who "require substantial food in liberal quantities" in order to replenish their exhausted energies (Woodward n.d.). Other psychiatrists also endorsed the differentiation of diet based on medical concerns, such as John B. Chapin, who advocated for the use of a "special dietary" for those patients who seemed the most likely to recover, in order to maximize their chances of cure (Chapin 1889: 14).

In practice, however, patients' social status generally offset other factors in determining their treatment. Most asylums that served both private and pauper patients reserved more diverse and high-quality diets for the former, and Worcester was no exception. While it may have been true that during Woodward's tenure "little distinction" was made in patients' diets, by 1902 the trustees—faced with accusations that the food served at the hospital was substandard—were forced to admit that "all private patients paying over $5 have a special diet" (Annual Report 1902: 20). Furthermore, upper- and middle-class patients were more likely to benefit from differentiation even when such differences were not directly tied to social rank or wealth. For instance, the privileging of patients based on "curability" tended to favor the middle and upper classes, who were generally viewed as more amenable to cure than their lower-class counterparts.

Classificatory systems based on merit were similarly likely to favor members of the native-born, Protestant middle class, whom psychiatrists viewed as hard-working and industrious, than paupers, who were typed as lazy and ignorant. A patient's refusal to work was viewed differently depending on his or her social class. While a pauper's refusal was viewed as evidence of laziness and moral weakness, in the upper class, it was viewed as the understandable expression of their refinement and delicacy. Furthermore, upper-class patients didn't need to work in order to gain access to the special treats offered as rewards to laborers, as they were often supplied with "luxuries" by friends and family members. In her letters to her brother, Mary E. Blanchard described the gifts she brought to their mother Sarah Seaver, a patient at McLean Asylum in the 1850s, including figs, brandy, strawberries, ice cream, and maple sugar, as well as a specially made cake and candy for her birthday (Blanchard 1854). Patients such as Sarah Seaver would have had a very different culinary experience from those whose families were unable or unwilling to supplement the asylum's diet with special treats.

THE ASYLUM FARM

A large portion of the food served at the Worcester State Hospital was grown on its farm, which was worked by patients. Under this system, patients served as both producers and consumers in a closed circuit that embodied the hospital's drive toward self-sufficiency—at least in theory. A sequence of patient labor linked the initial planting of produce to its harvesting, preparation, and finally serving. According to administrators, this labor was primarily therapeutic in nature, with its contribution to the hospital economy constituting a secondary benefit.

In the 1847 annual report, Woodward attempted to reconcile an apparent contradiction in psychiatric theory: namely, if it was true (as psychiatrists claimed) that "healthful agricultural employment . . . [was] one of the best restoratives" for the insane, why was it that farmers were the most heavily represented occupation among the male patients in the Worcester State Hospital (Annual Report 1838: 60)? Shouldn't these men, who were daily involved in an activity that was considered conducive to mental health, possess immunity from insanity? Woodward explained that while "moderate outdoor labor" was beneficial, economic demands forced farmers to work "too constantly and severely" for "small remuneration, leading to "overexertion . . . to supply the artificial wants created by the present state of society" (Annual Report 1847: 42). While the hospital could offer a temporary reprieve, it could not address the systemic problems that caused farmers to overwork in the first place. Woodward didn't explain what would happen to such patients when they were released and forced to resume their exhausting occupations. According to Pliny Earle's study of the patients discharged from Worcester, many of these individuals suffered relapses that forced them to return to the asylum multiple times (Earle 1876).

In order to furnish the means for "moderate outdoor labor," the first Worcester State Hospital was equipped with a 60-acre farm (figure 5.1) (Annual Report 1838: 4). Driven by increasing economic needs, the farm was expanded to 75 acres in 1845 and to 100 acres in 1846 (Annual Report 1845: 5, 1846: 59). The establishment of the second hospital provided the

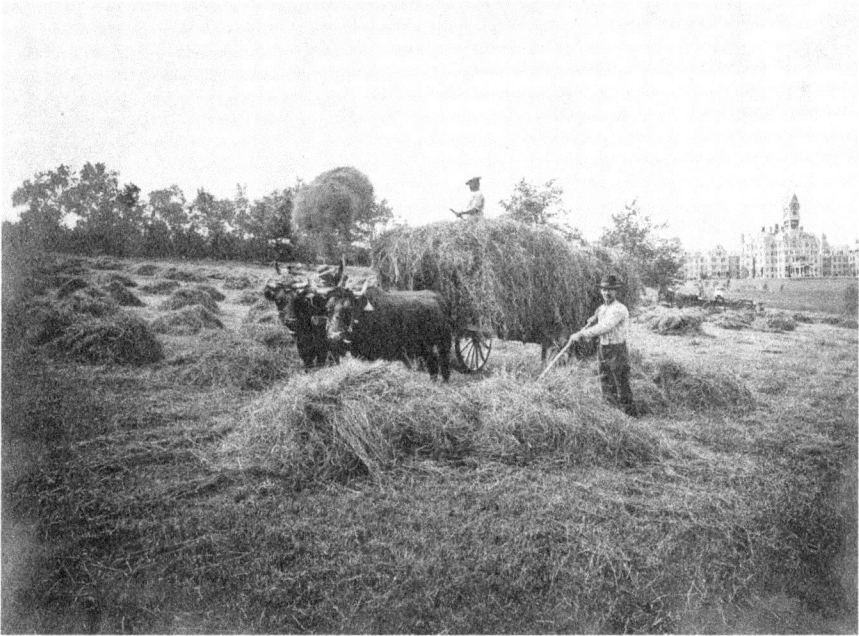

Figure 5.1   Patients Loading a Hay Wagon on the Asylum Farm, Circa 1880–1890.
This image shows the scope of the second hospital's agricultural fields, which extended southward from the main Kirkbride complex (in background). *Source*: Courtesy of the Worcester Historical Museum.

opportunity for an even greater expansion, encompassing 275 acres (Annual Report 1871: 8). In the 1890s, administrators constructed a large farmhouse, separate from the main Kirkbride complex, to accommodate the 50 patients who worked at the farm, along with their supervisor, his family, and other hired help (figure 5.2) (Annual Report 1894: 16). This model of separate accommodations for quiet and productive patients had been proposed decades earlier by Worcester superintendent Merrick Bemis, who had vigorously advocated for the adoption of the "cottage plan" rather than the linear style that was ultimately chosen for the second hospital. Bemis's vision was partially realized with the construction of the farmhouse; however, where Bemis had envisioned the cottage plan as a therapeutic instrument, it is evident that the farmhouse primarily served logistical and economic needs. The 50 patients selected for this work were described as "reasonably quiet and orderly, able to accomplish a certain amount of work on a farm." As a reward, they were given "greater freedom" and a "more liberal diet," which administrators hoped would incentivize good behavior among the other inmates of the hospital (Annual Report 1895: 5). The medical classification of patients thus overlapped with the hospital's specialization of labor as well as its system of

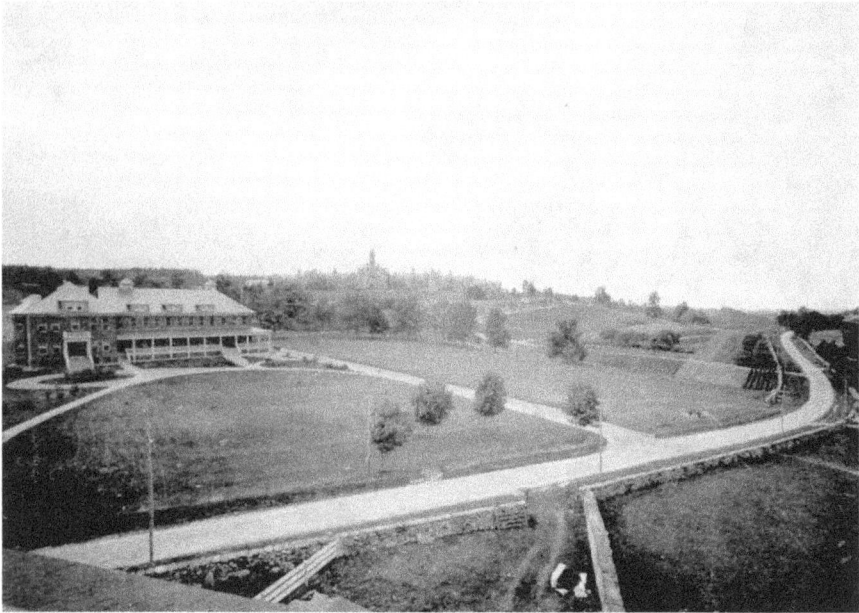

Figure 5.2　The Farmhouse of the Second Worcester State Hospital, Pictured in 1903, Was Built in the 1890s about a Quarter Mile Southeast of the Main Kirkbride Complex (Visible in Background). *Source*: Courtesy of the Harvard University Library.

rewards and punishments, reinforcing the connection between mental health, morality, and productivity.

Like the building itself, the second asylum farm became quickly insufficient to meet the demands of its population. In the first decade of the twentieth century, administrators secured the purchase of Hillside Farm, a 130-acre property in the neighboring town of Shrewsbury, to serve as an auxiliary "farm colony," providing a site for additional fields as well as accommodations for the hospital's cows and pigs (Annual Report 1912: 18). The effect of this addition was to segregate the hospital population even further, relegating its patient laborers to a space far beyond the observation of the hospital's administrators, the company of other patients, and the therapeutic resources of the main complex. Assuming that these resources actually offered curative potential, the removal of these productive but "incurable" patients from the main hospital might have served as a self-fulfilling prophecy, placing chronic patients into circumstances in which they were less likely to subvert the pessimistic prognosis they had been given.

The ideal of institutional self-sufficiency was ultimately unachievable. Administrators' commitment to the asylum farm as a self-sustaining source of agricultural produce meant that the hospital was subject to the vicissitudes

of the market, weather, and disease. Proceeds from sales of the hospital's produce declined during the Civil War, while periodic droughts forced the hospital to temporarily increase its dependence on exterior sources of food, driving
up expenditures (Annual Report 1865: 4). In 1915, the hospital's entire herd
of Holstein cattle was infected with hoof and mouth disease, necessitating
their slaughter (Annual Report 1915: 17). Although patients provided free
labor, they required the instruction and oversight of paid supervisors in order
to work effectively. Critics charged that the proceeds of asylum farms failed
to justify their existence. In 1902 Paul Mange, a farmer in nearby Millbury,
wrote to Rockwood Hoar, a trustee of the Worcester State Hospital, citing an
annual report that indicated the hospital farm "cost nearly $25,000 to run"
while producing "a return of only $4,000" (Mange 1902). Mange speculated
that the treasurer had failed to account for the value of the produce that had
been consumed at the hospital, such as milk and vegetables, and had recorded
as proceeds only the value of items that had been sold on the open market.

Scrutiny surrounding the economy of the hospital farm, and of the hospital in general, increased in the latter half of the nineteenth century, when
the apparent failure of asylums to realize the promises extended by the "cult
of curability" led the public to view their financial demands more critically.
State hospitals were, after all, dependent on state revenue for their continued
maintenance, and were therefore forced to justify their existence—if not
by the number of cures, then by their productivity. Having abandoned the
curative conceit, the Willard Asylum in Upstate New York adopted an institutional model predicated solely on the extraction of labor from its "incurable" inmates (Dwyer 1987). Because they were incurable, Willard's patient
population represented a stable and dependable source of labor. The labor
pool at Worcester was more capricious, as it included both acutely ill patients
who might recover within months as well as chronic cases who might remain
institutionalized for decades. It was this latter group of "incurables" who
were tapped to work the hospital farm, which expanded in accordance with
the growth of the overall patient population. The hospital's land holdings
peaked in the 1940s, when its agricultural properties encompassed 500 acres.
The farm ceased operations in the 1960s, after which much of the property
was parceled off and sold.

While David J. Myerson, Worcester's last superintendent, attributes the
end of the asylum farm to the decline in its economic viability, it may also
be attributed to the growing concern—which Myerson himself raises—that
"the major occupational programs in which patients participated met the
needs of the hospital, not the needs of the patient" (Myerson 1980: 100–101).
The mobilization of patients as unpaid laborers was increasingly viewed by
both the public and the psychiatric profession as exploitative and unethi-
cal. This shift in attitudes toward patient labor occurred in the context of

the emergence of anti-psychotic drugs, which for the first time offered the chance of meaningful recovery to a subset of patients who had been deemed incurably psychotic. The more likely patients were to recover, the less willing the public was to accept their relegation to a lifetime of unpaid drudgery. On a broader scale, the renewed hope of a cure (or at least a viable treatment) for mental illness and the reintegration of patients into the community undermined the perceived necessity for large, isolated residential institutions, which were increasingly seen as retrograde and abusive.

FORCED FEEDING: DOMINATION AND RESISTANCE

While psychiatrists were largely intolerant of social and class difference, they were even more hostile toward differences in perception and understanding that were associated with insanity, viewing these symptoms as expressions of deviance. In his memoir, Clifford Beers attempts to make his delusions legible to the reader, making the case that insanity possesses its own internal logic. One of Beers's delusions was the belief that he was being poisoned, a suspicion that seemed to be corroborated by the fact that "[n]one of [his] food [had] its natural flavor" (Beers 1913: 15). As a result, Beers refused the medicine that was offered to him in the asylum:

> To ask a patient in my condition to take a little medicated sugar seemed reasonable. But from my point of view my refusal was justifiable. That innocuous sugar disc to me seemed saturated with the blood of loved ones; and so much as to touch it was to shed their blood. (Ibid.)

Like the hymns of the hospital chapel—which he perceived as "funeral dirges"—the significance of these medicines was warped through the lens of Beers's illness, transforming intended agencies of cure into instruments of torture. Psychiatrists' efforts in mobilizing these agencies foundered not because of their failure to select a sufficiently uplifting hymn or to measure the correct dose of medicine, but because they refused to consider the patient's "point of view," through which seemingly irrational actions were "justifiable." After all, according to psychiatrists, taste—along with all other senses—ought to be uniform between individuals as a result of their shared human physiology. If the patient's sensory perceptions deviated from that objective standard, it was the psychiatrist's task not to accommodate that deviance, but to discipline it into conformity.

Even if patients didn't believe they were being intentionally poisoned, many reported that the medicines they were administered had negative effects. In a letter to trustee Rockwood Hoar, former Worcester patient

Arthur M. Sanborn stated that "the drugs that were introduced into my food and drink [in the hospital] had a partial effect on me, and raised a fever that ran for several weeks" (Sanborn 1898). Woodward wrote in an 1833 letter to Horace Mann that a patient had accused the superintendent of "[giving] him medicine to reduce his thought, in his food" (Woodward 1833). Although Woodward may not have done so, many psychiatrists endorsed the practice of surreptitiously dosing patients. In his treatise on hysteria, S. Weir Mitchell recommended that physicians whose patients resisted the medicinal use of iron powder should secretly introduce the powder to the patients' food in order to prove that "iron is not so difficult to take as [the patients] have been led to believe" (Mitchell 1877: 79–80). Other psychiatrists, such as Browne, objected to what they viewed as a violation of the patient's trust, claiming that dosing patients without their knowledge or consent gave truth to their paranoid suspicions (Browne 1875: 314).

For many patients, the refusal to eat might offer their only recourse against surreptitious dosing (whether real or imagined) or the severe side effects of medicines, as well as their most powerful means of protest against their confinement. Yet psychiatrists uniformly viewed the refusal to eat as a symptom of insanity, and furthermore, a symptom that must be overcome with physical force. The forced feeding of patients was not without controversy in the psychiatric community. In his 1838 treatise, William Ellis wrote that forced feeding was always unnecessary, as "the patient may be brought to acquiesce by management and skill" (Ellis 1838). Browne believed that only a small minority of patients necessitated forced feeding, stating that in his experience, "one ninth of the insane refuse food; in one thirtieth of these, the refusal could not be overcome" (Browne 1875: 305–306). Prior to resorting to force, psychiatrists should appeal to "moral and physical means," such as "bribes, commands, [and] entreaties," to convince patients to eat. For patients who feared being poisoned, psychiatrists should offer foods that were resistant to tampering (such as whole eggs, fruits, and nuts) (ibid.: 318–319).

Over time, psychiatrists' confidence in their ability to gain the trust and cooperation of the patient declined. Gerald Grob has attributed this tendency partly to the changing patient demographic in asylums, postulating that the influx of immigrants and paupers made it more difficult for psychiatrists to identify with their patients (Grob 1966). This lack of a common social footing, along with the belief that these patients were more resistant to treatment and guilty of immoral behavior, may have influenced medical practices and lowered the threshold at which psychiatrists resorted to force. By the mid-nineteenth century, the debate surrounding forced feeding increasingly focused upon when and how the act should be carried out, and not whether it represented the most effective or humane solution. In this way, the discourse surrounding forced feeding resembled that surrounding mechanical restraint, which was purportedly reduced or even eliminated in many asylums in the early nineteenth century, only to be reinstated in new, more "modern" forms (including that of chemical restraint) later in the century.

As in the case of mechanical restraint, psychiatrists' recourse to forced feeding was a source of embarrassment for the discipline because it revealed the failure of moral treatment to achieve one of its fundamental aims: to secure the cooperation of the patient by means of humane care and gentle persuasion. Yet psychiatrists who used forced feeding believed they had no alternative, as "a medical practitioner who allows a patient to thus commit suicide would deserve the utmost penalties" (Bell 1850). Forced feeding was thus viewed as necessary to maintain the life and well-being of the patient, but it was not without risk. The forced application of a naso-esophageal tube could and did result in the injury and death of patients (Browne 1875: 333). Yet even Browne considered the death of a patient as a result of forced feeding a "misadventure" rather than a travesty, justifying the use of the procedure on the grounds that feeding the patient—by any means necessary—was an essential element of treatment, without which the patient would not recover:

> If nutritious/abundant supplies of food constitute the most trustworthy remedy/ powerful auxiliary in the management of the insane, it must be obvious that the diminution or withdrawal of suitable aliment is calculated, not merely to retard and arrest recovery, but to multiple the causes of the condition upon which the mental phenomena depend. (Ibid.: 305)

Psychiatrists debated over the length of time that should be allowed to elapse before forced feeding was implemented. Like mechanical restraint, forced feeding was regarded—in theory—as an instrument of last resort, to be used only when the patient's survival was in jeopardy. Yet like mechanical restraint, it is evident that in the context of the overburdened, poorly staffed asylum, the expedience of forced feeding made it a more appealing alternative to the investment of time and energy that was necessary to earn the trust of an uncooperative patient. Although Browne advised psychiatrists to be conservative in the use of forced feeding, he estimated that the practice had been used in his own asylum "9,000 times" over the course of his 26-year superintendence at the Crichton Royal Asylum (ibid.: 331).

Furthermore, Browne described forced feeding not only as a form of medical treatment but as a psychological tactic used to secure the psychiatrist's dominance, stating that "[a] single introduction [of forced feeding] has often proved sufficient to convince patients of their utter helplessness, of the uselessness of obduracy" (ibid.). Similarly, Luther Bell stated that "the sight of the syringe may not always fail to be a turning argument" in convincing the patient to eat (Bell 1850: 230). Some patients, however, refused to yield in spite of the pain and trauma of forced feeding. Browne stated—with a perverse sort of pride—that one patient in the Crichton Asylum had been "supported by artificial alimentation" for more than two years (Browne 1875: 335), while Bell reported that several patients at McLean had been force-fed for periods ranging from 18 to 24 months (Bell 1850: 233). The procedure that psychiatrists claimed to use only as a last resort in the most extreme situations had thus been ensconced as a part of everyday care for certain patients. Even those patients who were not subject to forced feeding would have become familiar with the procedure through its use in others. Ebenezer Haskell witnessed the forced feeding of a fellow patient who subsequently told Haskell "he could not stand the torture again" and that "death was preferable to life" (Haskell 1868: 45). Shortly thereafter, the patient threw himself out of a window and died.

In describing their use of both forced feeding and mechanical restraint, psychiatrists cultivated a narrative of increasingly modern and humane treatment that served to soften the violence and trauma associated with these procedures. In doing so, they obfuscated the fact that many practices used by previous generations in the treatment of the insane—practices that early mental health reformers had decried as obscenely retrograde and barbaric—continued to be implemented in the modern asylum, albeit in slightly altered forms. In an article on forced feeding in the *American Journal of Insanity*, Bell described the instruments of forced feeding used in previous decades, including spouted vessels, iron tunnels, and wooden spoons, which often had the unintended effect of knocking out patients' teeth (ibid.: 227). In comparison, Bell presented the use of the naso-esophageal tube as modern and humane, despite the fact that it could—and did—result in the injury and death of patients. Bell suggested that his fellow psychiatrists "select the method which *appears* the least coarse and violent" (emphasis original), a curious choice of phrasing that seems to imply that it was more important to maintain the appearance of humane treatment rather than to secure the comfort and safety of the patient.

Psychiatrists legitimized the use of the naso-esophageal tube on the basis that the refusal to eat was symptomatic of an "active delusion" that must be treated (ibid.). Yet psychiatrists were aware that abstinence from food held social and cultural meanings that were separate from mental pathology, such as the practice of fasting among "religious ascetics" (Browne 1875: 308). In drawing an explicit connection between these ascetics and patients who were "impressed with the idea they are to fast for a definite period, in consequence of an immediate, supernatural communication," Browne made a gesture toward cultural relativism, entertaining the possibility that behaviors that were read as "symptoms" by psychiatrists might be interpreted differently in other contexts and by other individuals (ibid.).

Yet even if psychiatrists acknowledged that different standards of behavior existed, their actions reflected the assumption that *their* standard was the correct one.

As subjects of the asylum's all-encompassing disciplinary regime, patients possessed few means of registering their complaints and asserting their agency. Whether motivated by "active delusion" or not, the refusal to eat provided a means by which patients could circumvent the hospital's control over their bodies and thereby reclaim it for themselves. In describing this refusal a "case of pure will," Bell revealed how forced feeding was mobilized as a weapon in the battle between psychiatrist and patient (Bell 1850: 227). While psychiatrists may have believed that the patient was delusional, they nonetheless acknowledged that the patient *had* agency and was capable of exerting it in defiance of institutional dominance. The habitual use of forced feeding suggests that this defiance was seen as more threatening to the institutional order than the delusion itself. After all, delusions were located in the patient's mind; it was only when they came into active confrontation with the authority of the superintendent that they became problematic and therefore required intervention.

TEA PARTIES

The practice of dining at the Worcester State Hospital was conceptualized as an instrument within its moral program, which could be used to inculcate certain forms of behavior and even transform character. As Woodward wrote, "[t]he difference between eating food in solitude from a tin or wooden dish with the fingers or a spoon, and going to a neatly furnished table, and taking meals from crockery with a knife and fork, is the difference between a savage and a civilized man" (Annual Report 1839: 95). In this statement, "savagery" is coded as insanity; to be civilized is to become sane. Yet the prevailing medical discourse described insanity as a "disease of civilization," to which savages were virtually immune. According to psychiatrists, civilization had caused the patient's insanity, turning a sane man into an irrational savage. To be cured, he must enter the asylum, a "technological marvel" unique to modern civilization, where he would eat like a savage, but dine like a gentleman; eschew the pleasures of civilization while meeting its economic needs; return to a state of nature while being educated in bourgeois manners and values. Patients caught in this system could not be blamed for wondering exactly what kind of person the asylum wanted them to be.

The role played by tea in the asylum is representative of this dissonance, occupying a fraught position along the boundary between gentility and vice. Psychiatrists claimed the responsibility for policing this boundary, but didn't always agree on its definition. Pliny Earle believed that the insane should avoid tea and coffee. Similarly, Black wrote that that although "[t]ea, coffee, and tobacco don't stimulate with the effects of opium and liquors," they "prepare the way by developing the desire for stimulation" (Black 1873: 124). Woodward disagreed, stating that "tea, coffee, and milk are used liberally in the Hospital," with positive results (Annual Report 1836: 185). Furthermore, the consumption of tea provided the opportunity to exert a moral influence over the patient. Because the insane were believed to have been reduced to the level of savages, the tea party—and dining in general—acted as an arena in which patients could practice the arts of gentility. The ability to successfully perform social rituals such as tea drinking was treated as an index of mental health. A sane person demonstrated not only the capacity to enjoy the refinements of civilization, but to maintain self-control, which prevented the pursuit of pleasure from devolving into pathological overindulgence.

Woodward boasted that at the Worcester State Hospital, "[t]ables were set neatly, furnished with knives, forks, and crockery. We have at no time half a dozen patients who cannot go to the table and eat with knives and forks" (Annual Report 1839: 95)—statements that were intended to prove the efficacy of the hospital in civilizing (and thus curing) its patients. He wrote that the majority of patients "conduct[ed] themselves with decorum" at the table (Annual Report 1838: 59).

It is illustrative that the therapeutic efficacy of the hospital was couched in terms of teapots, crockery, and the "decorum" that patients displayed in using them. Mental health was still largely coterminous with a specific type of social fluency; sanity was articulated in terms of external behavior—that is, the ability to play one's part at a tea party—rather than internal thoughts and feelings. Furthermore, the moral program that was intended to instill patients with the "decorum" and restraint appropriate to a tea party represented part of the larger institutional project to remake the insane into useful, genteel citizens. Etiquette, along with time-keeping and the production of labor, was one of the many disciplines that drove the ideological machinery of capitalism (Leone 1999: 196). Through a series of discursive maneuvers that reinscribed the authority of God into that of a scientifically objective "Nature," these historically contingent codes of behavior were embedded into standards of mental health.

The objective of institutional discipline was to compel patients to internalize these codes, thus rendering physical force unnecessary. Accordingly, psychiatrists were keen to demonstrate the efficacy of the disciplinary function of the asylum by claiming that the insane were trusted with the use of crockery and even knives. This trust formed a central part of the bonds of "confidence" between psychiatrist and patient that were thought to be essential for recovery (Tomes 1984). Yet psychiatrists' confidence in the insane was rarely unqualified. As described by Conolly, the knives used by patients at the Hanwell Asylum were "only sharpened along a portion of [their] edge," and the forks had "very short prongs" (Conolly 1847: 75). Accordingly, the objects that were intended to prove the asylum's trust in its patients may have had the opposite effect, serving—much like its barred windows—as potent reminders of their confinement.

Similarly, despite Woodward's portrayal of perfect "decorum" among his patients, the *System of Regulations* used during his tenure suggests that meals were heavily choreographed and dependent on the supervision and intervention of attendants: "one Attendant must always be present at the meals, carve the food and distribute it to such as are no competent to do it for themselves, and see that each one has his proper supply. He must also be careful that no knife, fork, or other article, be carried from the table by the patients" ("System of regulations" 1833: 13). Such regulations speak to the potential for violence that administrators and superintendents tended to downplay in their reports, but that represented a daily reality for attendants and patients. For many patients, the attempt to practice genteel modes of dining may have struck a discordant note in the context of the asylum, which patients' accounts describe as volatile, disorderly, and shockingly foreign to those unaccustomed to institutional life.

The therapeutic asylum was formed on the premise that the insane, despite their illness, were human beings who were capable of being restored. The modern campaign of moral treatment was traced to Philippe Pinel's apocryphal removal of the chains from the women at the Salpêtrière Asylum. The introduction of cutlery and crockery served a similarly discursive purpose in embodying the aims of moral treatment as a humane and humanizing project. It is no coincidence that upon his arrival at the Pennsylvania Hospital for the Insane as its new superintendent, the first actions taken by Thomas Story Kirkbride were to remove restraints and to construct a "regular dining room" with "ordinary utensils and crockery," all of which had been "unknown in the old institution" (Tomes 1984: 19). A similar and equally symbolic transformation took place at Hanwell, where Conolly gradually replaced metal plates with ceramic pieces, proudly reporting that "breakage is insignificant" (Conolly 1847: 75). The use of crockery thus came to assume particular significance as a symbol of the humanity of lunatics and the hope for their recovery in the new therapeutic asylum.

It is meaningful that dining etiquette in particular was invested with this symbolic import. In the nineteenth century, "the middle classes adopted 'table manners' as a new discriminatory code" (Hamilakis 2014: 23). As a result, "[e]ating lost part of [its] sensuous, experiential value, and became more like a theatre, a performance where one should be constantly conscious of the image one projects" (ibid.). This performance was mobilized in psychiatry as both a means of cure and standard for recovery. Sets of dishes and eating utensils were among those objects that Paul Shackel identifies as "items associated with people who saw themselves as individuals . . . use to demonstrate merit, punctuality, cleanliness, numeracy, manners, literacy, and other rationalized traits important to modern notions of productivity" (Shackel 1993). Such values were deeply embedded in discourses surrounding sanity and madness.

Psychiatrists' descriptions of the "disease of civilization" suggest that the recent rise in the incidence of insanity was threatening not because of lunatics' personal suffering or the danger they posed to others, but due to the loss of their labor in a society that couched human value in terms of productivity. Insanity removed the individual "from the sphere of action and usefulness," causing "the loss of productive power to families and the State" and "add[ing] to public and private burdens" ("Insanity in Massachusetts" 1861: 94–95). In 1849, Woodward boasted that as a result of their tenure in the hospital, "[m]any valuable citizens . . . have been restored to happiness and usefulness in society" (Annual Report 1849: 4). For this reason, the ability of the chronic insane to perform "useful" labor in an asylum was viewed as an acceptable outcome when it was acknowledged that not all patients could be cured.

The investment of bourgeois values into standards of mental health meant that not all patients were equally equipped to meet the hospital's standards, a fact that no doubt contributed to the accumulation of "incurables." Psychiatrists' perception that the lower classes were less likely to recover was correct, albeit not for the reasons that they claimed. Through no fault of their own, lower-class patients had a distinct experience of asylum life, characterized by a lower quality of accommodations and diet, a greater amount of labor, and less personalized attention from psychiatrists respective to their middle- and upper-class counterparts. Superintendents admitted that they devoted more time and effort toward those patients they viewed as likely to recover: a group that inevitably included more native-born and upper-class patients than paupers and immigrants.

At many asylums, including Worcester, certain patients were invited to dine with the superintendent's family, a gesture that was intended to build their foundation of trust. According to Morrill Wyman, the son of the first superintendent of the McLean Asylum, his father had "one or more boarders [patients] always at [his] table," who "had rooms in the mansion house and mingled with the family" (Little 1972: 43). Yet what was presented as an equalizing and progressive gesture was, in fact, a practice that served to further reinforce inequalities. These inequalities might have been less pronounced at private asylums such as McLean, in which most patients belonged to the upper and middle classes. At state hospitals such as Worcester, however, the superintendents' selection likely contributed to the divide between upper- and middle-class patients and paupers.

During her first few months at the Jacksonville Asylum, Elizabeth Packard was among the patients favored by the superintendent's attention. Along with eating at his table, she was given a well-furnished room, access to her possessions, and the freedom to "read, knit, sew, ride, and walk" as she pleased (Packard 1873: 101). Packard would have made an ideal dinner companion for the superintendent: the daughter and wife of ministers, she was well educated and articulate; furthermore, according to the later verdict of the state supreme court, she was not insane. Yet even Packard's invitation was contingent on her continued deference to the superintendent; after she first openly criticized the institution, her privileges were revoked and she was relocated to the violent ward. "[D]ining with the insane," she wrote, "I must confess, I did feel more out of my proper place, than I had while in the reception room of refined society" (ibid.: 81). Like psychiatrists, Packard regarded insanity and refinement as antonyms, conflating social class and mental status. Hill made a similar statement about the mortifying experience of her association with the insane, specifically having "to eat the same food, so poor!" and "to drink the same drink" (Hill 1881: 34).

For those patients who were not invited to the superintendent's table, dining in the asylum was a decidedly different experience. The patients confined to Worcester's strong rooms ate without furniture or utensils, their food delivered via an "aperture" in their cells (Annual Report 1854: 26). Furthermore, the logistics surrounding dining at the hospital changed radically over time and was heavily impacted by the growth of its patient population. In the first hospital, dining rooms were located in each story of the building, served from external kitchens by dumbwaiters (figure 5.3) (Annual Report 1844: 13). In the second hospital, a track running through the hospital basement allowed the distribution of food from a centralized kitchen to dining rooms in each ward (Annual Report 1879: 15). Yet these new dining rooms were quickly rendered obsolete by the increasing number of patients and changing standards for dining service. Trustees complained of the difficulty of serving patients in the "numerous small, unattractive dining rooms, many [of which were] distant from the kitchen" (Annual Report 1915: 8). By 1904, more than a third of the hospital's patient population was being "served on trays in the wards" for want of space. Later on, tables were crammed into the corridors to meet the need for seating during meals (Annual Report 1912: 8).

Writing to Joseph Parish in 1845, Woodward had expressed his preference for small dining rooms over larger ones that mixed residents from multiple wards, stating that the latter compromised classification, exposing "the quiet convalescent patients" to those who were "excited" and "unattuned to habits

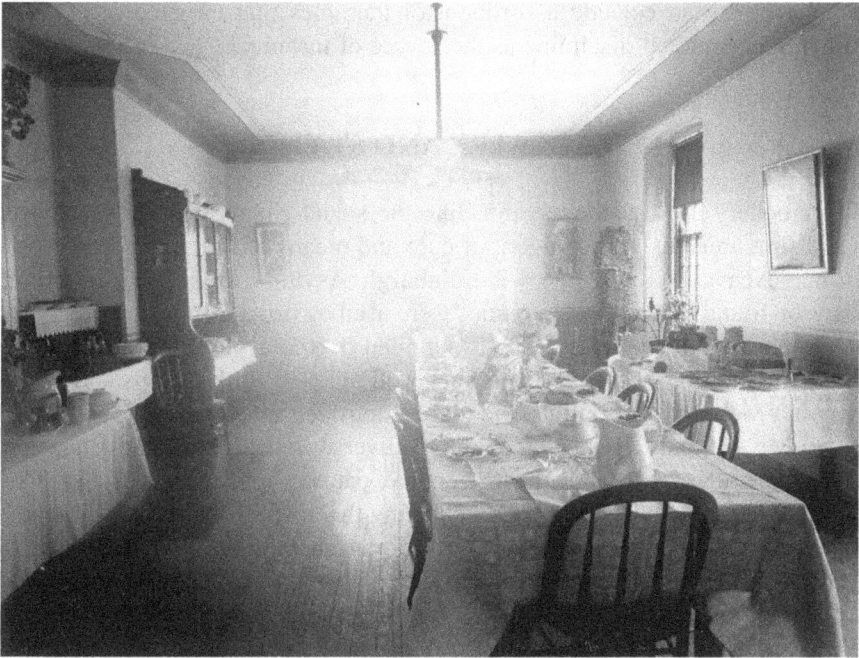

Figure 5.3   A Dining Room in the Second Worcester State Hospital, Prior to the Implementation of a Cafeteria System, Circa 1870s–1920s. *Source*: Courtesy of the Worcester Historical Museum.

of cleanliness and order." "In those small dining rooms those only who are in daily habits of associating come together," he wrote, which helped promote good feelings and behavior between patients (Woodward 1845). Many of Woodward's interventions at the Worcester State Hospital aimed at normalizing the experience of patients in accordance with his own ideas of domestic gentility. This included the taking of meals with known associates of similar comportment and background. To Woodward, the superintendent's control over every facet of patient dining—from the organization of diners to the type of food and the way it was served—was justified by the fact that insanity was thought to stem from the patient's poor choices. In order to recover, the patient must temporarily relinquish the power of decision-making to the superintendent, who would act as a paternal figure and moral educator until the patient was well enough to exert self-discipline. By the early twentieth century, mental illness was increasingly attributed to inheritance and physiological defects that were beyond the patient's control. Under this model of mental disorder, the significance of dining as a remedial measure declined. While social fluency was still used as an index of recovery and the efficacy of institutional order, the holistic program of moral treatment would be supplanted by an eclectic assortment of therapies that targeted physiology rather than personal discipline as the source of insanity.

CROCKERY AND STATUS

The crockery used at the asylum, like the social rituals that surrounded it, acted simultaneously as an agent of cure and means of social differentiation. In her excavation at the Royal Edinburgh Asylum, archaeologist Joanna Dawson found that distinct ceramics were used by private and pauper patients (Dawson 2003). The coarse bowls supplied by the asylum to paupers were "all-purpose food vessel[s]" that were well adapted to the soups and gruels that they were fed. In contrast, the more extensive range of crockery afforded to private patients reflected their more diverse and higher quality cuisine. Over the course of the nineteenth century, paupers' crockery was expanded to include soup and dessert plates, reflecting the diversification of their menu. When the asylum switched from its Edinburgh pottery supplier to one in Staffordshire, they adopted a color code. Gold-rimmed pieces were reserved for private patients, while those of "humbler rank" were given pottery with blue, red, and pink rims, possibly corresponding to the different wards occupied by paupers (ibid.: 46).

In her archaeological study of the Magdalen Society in Philadelphia, Lu Ann De Cunzo discovered that crockery served not only to differentiate among its inmates but also to distinguish between these "fallen women" and their white, middle-class overseers. While inmates were supplied with mismatched, old-fashioned, and inexpensive crockery, overseers used uniform ceramic sets of relatively high value, a distinction which served both to "express a sense of group identity" among these bourgeois women and to "reinforc[e] [their] differentness" from their lower-class charges (De Cunzo 1995: 74). According to Suzanne Spencer-Wood, most nineteenth-century institutions across the Northeast United States supplied their inmates with "uniform tinware or white ceramics," suited for the consumption of the "lowest cost food," a measure that served both economical and ideological needs (Spencer-Wood 2010). The whiteness, durability, and uniformity of institutional ceramics served as material embodiments of the hospital's moral and medical program.

In contrast to the distinctly institutional-style white ceramics that have been noted in archaeological studies of nineteenth-century institutions, the ceramics purchased for the Worcester State Hospital at the time of its establishment—as documented in a collection of receipts (table 5.1)—include a variety of feather-edged and transfer-printed pieces, which would have been markedly decorative, colorful, and delicate. Furthermore, unlike the

Table 5.1   **Tablewares Purchased for the Worcester State Hospital, 1833**

Item	Amount	Price	Vendor
Plates 2nd size 45	3 doz.	$1.35	Rice & Sweetser
Plates 3rd size 37	3 doz.	$1.11	Rice & Sweetser
Plates 4th size 29	3 doz.	$0.87	Rice & Sweetser
Tray	1	$0.07	Henry Wheeler
Wooden spoons	5	$0.40	Henry Wheeler
Planished tin coffee pot	1	$1.75	Henry W. Miller, Worcester
Tin tea canisters	2	$0.60	Henry W. Miller, Worcester
Square tin pans	6	$0.83	Henry W. Miller, Worcester
½ pt col mugs	6 doz.	$2.88	Rice & Sweetser
½ qt col bowls	4 doz.	$4.80	Rice & Sweetser
½ pt col bowls	4 doz.	$3.36	Rice & Sweetser
Sets col teas	24	$3.60	Rice & Sweetser
Pitchers	24	$1.68	Rice & Sweetser
16 in edged dishes	12	$9.30	Rice & Sweetser
12 in edged dishes	24	$3.00	Rice & Sweetser
12 in edged nappie[?]	24	$9.72	Rice & Sweetser
24 8 in edged nappie[?]	24	$2.40	Rice & Sweetser
12 qt cc bowls rimd		$0.96	Rice & Sweetser
Col jugs or pitchers	12	$2.40	Rice & Sweetser
2 qt bowls	6	$0.90	Rice & Sweetser
Soy[?] mugs	1 doz.	$0.48	Rice & Sweetser
Tavern tumblers	1 doz.	$0.83	Rice & Sweetser
Knives and forks	½ gro	$5.00	George T. Rice & Co.
Plates and c.	6	$1.00	Leonard Poole
Deep blue-printed plates	1 dozen	$1.12	William H. Swan, Worcester
One printed soup tureen and four pr woolen stockings		$4.21	William H. Swan
Small fancy mugs	1 dozen	$0.45	William H. Swan, Worcester
Small mugs	2 5/12 dozen	$1.41	William H. Swan, Worcester
Plates	4 dozen	$1.80	Rice & Sweetser
6 pitchers and 48 C.C. pt mugs		$2.88	Rice & Sweetser
Coffee leach[?] & pot		$5.00	C. Newcomb, Worcester
Coffee roaster		$5.50	C. Newcomb, Worcester
Coffee pots	2	$1.33	C. Newcomb, Worcester
Coffee pot	1	$0.67	C. Newcomb, Worcester
Cake cutter		$0.12	C. Newcomb, Worcester
Coffee pots	3	$2.00	C. Newcomb, Worcester
Ladles	6	$0.75	C. Newcomb, Worcester
Tea kettle and strainer		$2.00	C. Newcomb, Worcester

(Continued)

Table 5.1   Tablewares Purchased for the Worcester State Hospital, 1833 (*Continued*)

Item	Amount	Price	Vendor
Cast iron kettle and bailing		$1.25	Henry W. Miller
½ gross knives and forks and 3 doz. spoons		$7.88	George T. Rice & Co., Worcester
2 dozen spoons 1 drudging box		$1.65	George T. Rice & Co., Worcester
Knives and forks	½ gross	$5.50	George T. Rice & Co., Worcester
Soup plates	3 dozen	$1.75	Rice & Sweetser
Plates	2 dozen	$1.17	Rice & Sweetser
First size plates	24	$2.25	Charles P. Hitchcock
Second size plates	23	$1.92	Charles P. Hitchcock
Third size plates	22	$1.61	Charles P. Hitchcock
Fourth size plates	23	$1.44	Charles P. Hitchcock
Fifth size plates	24	$1.25	Charles P. Hitchcock
Sixth size plates	21	$0.87	Charles P. Hitchcock
20 inch platter	1	$1.62	Charles P. Hitchcock
16 inch platters	2	$2.16	Charles P. Hitchcock
12 inch platters	4	$2.00	Charles P. Hitchcock
10 inch platters	2	$0.67	Charles P. Hitchcock
9 inch platters	2	$0.50	Charles P. Hitchcock
Covered dishes	2	$1.83	Charles P. Hitchcock
Oval dishes	2	$1.00	Charles P. Hitchcock
Sauce tureens	2	$1.83	Charles P. Hitchcock
Coffee cups and saucers	12	$1.75	Charles P. Hitchcock
Tea cups and saucers	11	$0.75	Charles P. Hitchcock
Teapots	2	$0.75	Charles P. Hitchcock
Large bowls	2	$0.33	Charles P. Hitchcock
Bowls	2	$0.25	Charles P. Hitchcock
Sugar bowl	1	$0.29	Charles P. Hitchcock
Cream pitcher	1	$0.20	Charles P. Hitchcock
Knives and forks	½ gross	$5.00	George T. Rice & Co., Worcester
Steel top'd knives and forks	3 cases	$4.50	George T. Rice & Co., Worcester
Steep top'd carving knife and fork	1	$0.08	George T. Rice & Co., Worcester
Britannia table spoons	½ gross	$4.50	George T. Rice & Co., Worcester
Britannia tea spoons	¾ gross	$2.62	George T. Rice & Co., Worcester
Bread knives	½ dozen	$1.30	George T. Rice & Co., Worcester
Bread knives	1/6 dozen	$0.70	George T. Rice & Co., Worcester
Three pint tin teapots	2	$0.67	George T. Rice & Co., Worcester

(*Continued*)

Table 5.1   Tablewares Purchased for the Worcester State Hospital, 1833 (*Continued*)

Item	Amount	Price	Vendor
Carving knives & forks	½ dozen	$3.25	George T. Rice & Co., Worcester
Bread trays	5/6 dozen	$2.7	George T. Rice & Co., Worcester
Coffee mill		$0.87	George T. Rice & Co., Worcester
28 in tea waiters [?]	½ dozen	$4.50	George T. Rice & Co., Worcester
Tin sauce pan		$1.12	George T. Rice & Co., Worcester
Tin sauce pans	2	$1.80	George T. Rice & Co., Worcester
Brass kettle		$3.78	George T. Rice & Co., Worcester
Iron kettle		$2.00	George T. Rice & Co., Worcester
Coffee mill		$0.8[cutoff]	George T. Rice & Co., Worcester
Tea boiler		$4.12	George T. Rice & Co., Worcester
One padlock, One iron kettle, wire		$0.36	Henry W. Miller
Planished tin coffeepots	2	$1.75	Henry W. Miller
Tea canisters	2	$0.60	Henry W. Miller

Compiled from State Lunatic Hospital Filings, Massachusetts State Archives, Boston, Mass.

ceramics at the Magdalen Society, they were purchased in matching sets. The "deep blue printed plates" purchased from local merchant William H. Swan may have included the kinds of Romantic or exotic scenes commonly found in transfer-printed plates of this period. John R. Haddad describes how such scenes served as "magical portal[s]" into imagined worlds for the Americans who viewed them, particularly women and girls who were circumscribed within the domestic sphere (Haddad 2007). At the time of the hospital's creation, such scenes might have been envisioned as aesthetically and ideologically consonant with the Romantic paradigm underlying the institution and its efforts to create a rural idyll. In practice, they might have provided a means of escape from the monotonous uniformity of the institution, similar to the artwork that were used to "beautify" the walls of the galleries. According to administrators, these images served to "give the appearance of life and gaiety" and "relieve the wards of their cheerless, sober look" (Annual Report 1856: 49).

While the quality of the ceramics purchased for the Worcester State Hospital conjures a different vision of institutional life than the standardized white china found at other institutions, this difference may reflect the vagaries of preservation and changing institutional practices over time rather than a distinctive approach on the part of its administrators. These receipts represent a time before the hardy, white, semi-vitrified ceramics favored by institutions—known as white granite or ironstone—became widely available (Godden 1999; Wetherbee 1985). Accordingly, administrators simply purchased large quantities of the ceramics that were produced and sold for a domestic market. One of the first institutions of its kind, and the only one in Massachusetts for several decades, the Worcester State Hospital was established before the market for institutional ceramics existed. Accordingly, rather than buying all of the ceramics needed for the several hundred patients and staff of the hospital at once, they were forced to purchase them in quantities of one to four dozen, from several different stores in Worcester. Over time, with the expansion of institutions in the United States, American ceramic manufacturers would emerge to meet the demand for large quantities of white, institutional-grade china, as they did in Edinburgh and Staffordshire to supply institutions such as the Royal Edinburgh Asylum (Dawson 2013). The receipts from the first Worcester State Hospital suggest that administrators were no less concerned with frugality than their counterparts at other institutions; the "CC"—or creamware—mugs and bowls they selected represented the most inexpensive option for ceramics at the time (Miller 1991).

The use of crockery in the asylum would have had a particular effect in shaping the roles of women, who were considered the natural guardians of "domesticity and social reproduction" (Wall 1994: 111). In keeping with their duties outside of the institution, female patients in the asylum were responsible for undertaking the labor of preparing meals, setting and clearing the table, and performing the social rituals surrounding tea drinking. However, these patients lacked the agency and autonomy that women in the outside world were able to exercise despite the circumscribed limits of the domestic sphere. As Diana Wall writes, nineteenth-century women played a significant role as "social negotiators" who mobilized the consumption and use of ceramics to define and maintain the status of their families (ibid.). As part of this role, women held the authority to choose which ceramics the family would own and which sets they would use in different social contexts. In contrast, the ceramics at the Worcester State Hospital were not chosen by the women who used them, but by male administrators who would have lacked the insight into the social meanings and ritual functions of ceramics that were typically arbitrated by women. To these administrators, patients played a passive, rather than an active role in the transmission of values and negotiation of identities. As in every other sphere of the asylum, administrators assumed an attitude of paternalism in their management of the institution's ceramics, trusting that their judgment was inherently superior to that of their irrational and misguided charges (Porter 1985).

"A CHEAP IMITATION OF FOOD"

Despite the emphasis that psychiatrists placed on diet as an essential part of their remedial toolkit, the food that was served at state hospitals was widely criticized as nutritionally poor and strikingly unappetizing. Some of the most visceral and repugnant passages in Nelly Bly's 1887 exposé of conditions at the Blackwell's Island Hospital are those that describe the food she was forced to consume as a patient. Her first meal consisted of "a bowl of cold tea, a slice of buttered bread and a saucer of oatmeal, with molasses on it" (Bly 1887). The butter "was so horrible that one could not eat it"; the tea "had no sugar, and it tasted as if it had been made in copper," and the bread was "dirty" and "black" in color, "hard, and in places nothing more than dried dough," and contained a spider. Reflecting on her ten days in the asylum, Bly stated that "the eating was one of the most horrible things."

> Excepting the first two days after I entered the asylum, there was no salt for the food. The hungry and even famishing women made an attempt to eat the horrible messes. Mustard and vinegar were put on meat and in soup to give it a taste, but it only helped to make it worse. Even that was all consumed after two days, and the patients had to try to choke down fresh fish, just boiled in water, without salt, pepper or butter; mutton, beef and potatoes without the faintest seasoning. The most insane refused to swallow the food and were threatened with punishment. In our short walks we passed the kitchen where food was prepared for the nurses and doctors. There we got glimpses of melons and grapes and all kinds of fruits, beautiful white bread and nice meats, and the hungry feeling would be increased tenfold. I spoke to some of the physicians, but it had no effect, and when I was taken away the food was yet unsalted. (Bly 1887)

While recognizing her disgust, Bly's fellow patients urged her to eat, parroting the belief of contemporary psychiatrists that starvation was productive of mental disorder: "To have a good brain the stomach must be cared for" (Bly 1887). Ironically, this maxim—while embraced by both psychiatrists and patients—was impossible to follow in the asylum due to the poor quality of the food.

Elizabeth Packard was also critical of the cuisine served at the asylum. A disciple of health reformer Sylvester Graham, she was accustomed to a diet of

"Graham bread, fruits and vegetables," and feared that the "plain and coarse" meals she consumed at Jacksonville, consisting of "bolted bread and meat, tea and coffee," would cause her "health [to] materially suffer" (Packard 1873: 76). Furthermore, she complained that the food and drink served to patients in the violent ward—to which she was confined as a punishment for criticizing the superintendent—were "contaminated with the smell" of their filthy surroundings (ibid.: 116).

Although Pliny Earle—like most psychiatrists—considered good nutrition essential to recovery from insanity, a state investigation in 1870 found that the food served at his institution at Northampton was "badly cooked" and "often of bad quality" ("Report of a Committee . . ." 1870: 8). Similar complaints against the Worcester State Hospital came to a head in 1902, when the poor quality of its food served formed one of the central complaints cited in a widely publicized nurses' strike. The nurses claimed that the food served to patients was "rotten and foul-smelling," and that those who refused to eat it were punitively "force fed"—a statement that challenges psychiatrists' widely held claim that forced feeding was used exclusively as a measure of last resort upon psychotic and delusional patients ("Nurses in rebellion" 1902, "Put out bag and baggage!" 1902). If the claims of the nurses, and of Packard and Bly, regarding the quality of food served at state hospitals were correct, then patients' refusal to eat may be reconceptualized as a measure meant to protect their own well-being, and forced feeding as a direct assault against patients' health and autonomy.

Worcester trustees went to great lengths to repudiate the nurses' claims, publishing an account of the items that were grown on the hospital's farm and were thus provided "fresher than what could be obtained at the market," and obtaining testaments from their outside food suppliers to the quality and freshness of the food (Annual Report 1902). The trustees did concede that the hospital had recently adopted the use of oleomargarine—a newly developed butter substitute that the strikers called a "cheap imitation of food"—due to the prohibitive costs of butter. However, they insisted that the oleomargarine was perfectly edible, and was regularly consumed by administrators and trustees during their visits to the hospital without complaint (ibid.).

Despite the trustees' fervor in defending the hospital's dietary program, accounts from throughout the early twentieth century corroborate the charge that the hospital's food was sub-par. Furthermore, administrators admitted that they struggled to feed the growing patient population. In 1913, the hospital was dogged by another scandal surrounding the alleged waste of food. The hospital's matron, Mary Dudley, attributed the waste to the fact that patients "sometimes refuse to eat" ("Great waste of food at hospital" 1913). Notably, Dudley did not state that the patients' refusal was a symptom of their insanity; instead, she admitted that many patients "did not like the food," a grievance that she seemed to take seriously, as she forwarded their complaints to the chef (ibid.). During World War I, administrators strove to increase the institution's agricultural productivity in order to compensate for rations imposed on meat, sugar, and wheat (Annual Report 1917: 13, 1918: 16). Given the defects of the institutional diet, it is possible that at least part of the pathologies exhibited by patients were iatrogenic: diseases of institution-alization, caused directly by the conditions at the hospital. While originally conceptualized as an instrument of cure, the asylum diet—along with many other facets of treatment—had become a contributor to the very illnesses that it was intended to ameliorate.

CONCLUSION

Nineteenth-century psychiatrists ascribed to a model of health that was predicated on the existence of objective and strictly defined laws of nature. To these psychiatrists, illness—including insanity—was a manifestation of the individual's divergence from these "commandments."

The allegedly "natural" rules governing the production of consumption of food, however, were structured by a set of distinctively bourgeois moral values that demonized overindulgence and intemperance, encour-aged self-discipline and productivity, and treated gentility as an index of social worth—as well as of sanity. The perceived inability of the insane to meet bourgeois standards of gentility marked them not only as mentally disordered but also inferior and barbarous. This stigmatization was deepened by the fact that many of the asylum's patients belonged to the working or lower classes of society. Accordingly, the asylum acted not only as a therapeutic instrument but also as a moral machine that was designed to transform lazy, indolent transgressors into useful, "decorous" citizens. Because the theory and mechanics underlying this machine seemed straightforward and self-evident to psychiatrists, they were confounded when the asylum failed to translate its ideals into real-ity. While psychiatrists tended to blame this failure on the intractable immorality and weakness of individual patients, particularly paupers and immigrants, a review of the various meanings and uses of food in the hospital reveals the fault lines that ran through the asylum's ideological structure.

One of these fault lines can be traced to the dissonances of psychiatric theory, which treated socially and historically contingent values surrounding decorous behavior—including the ability to conduct oneself at a tea party and dine with "decorum"—as medical and scientific laws invested with a quasi-divine authority. As a result of their unfailing confidence in the existence of an objective standard of "Nature," as exhibited in personal behavior and values surrounding diet and dining, psychiatrists lacked the reflexivity and sensitivity toward difference that were necessary to provide patients from a wide variety of backgrounds with the sympathetic, individualized attention that moral treatment required. Instead of trying to understand patients on their own terms, psychiatrists viewed patients—particularly those who were uncooperative and unrefined—as deviants who needed to be corrected and opponents in a battle of wills. Patients who were faced with the all-encompassing and uncompromising force of the psychiatrist's authority responded with strategies that were intended to preserve their well-being and autonomy. The resulting dynamic of domination and resistance involved the use of coercive, violent, and punitive measures such as forced feeding. Psychiatrists' myopic focus on insanity as the explanation for any seemingly aberrant behavior prevented them from acknowledging legitimate complaints, respecting their patients' subjectivities, and questioning their own assumptions. Because the efficacy of the asylum—and, by extension, the psychiatric profession—was thought to hinge on the paternalistic and singular authority of its central authority figure, patients' acts of resistance were viewed not simply as expressions of insanity, but as threats to institutional order and to the legitimacy of psychiatry.

A second fault line can be traced to the core identity of the institution, which was founded upon paradoxical concepts of "Nature" and civilization. On the one hand, the nineteenth-century total institution was a product of modernity: a "technological marvel" that leveraged the latest discoveries in architecture, biomedicine, and social discipline (Yanni 2007). On the other hand, its therapeutic program was predicated on the reenactment of an idealized, mythologized agrarian past based upon an Edenic vision of Nature. The result was a Frankensteinian hybrid situated halfway between capitalist machine and feudal kingdom. While intentionally segregated from the world, the asylum was dependent on the nearest city for its population and resources, and upon state appropriations for the maintenance of its infrastructure. While purporting to offer the latest in medical therapeutics, psychiatrists in the asylum were radically segregated from their peers in medicine, which foreclosed communication and contributed to asylums' reputation as custodial and scientifically stagnant.

Patients bore the greatest burdens of the hospital's crisis of identity. They were charged with the work of capitalist laborers, yet denied the incentive of capital; instructed to act like proper citizens while being denied freedom, the defining feature of citizenship; subjected to a program of therapy that treated bourgeois values as irrefutable scientific facts; and expected to recover from insanity while being denied the full advantages of the therapeutic resources that the asylum promised. Their tenure at the hospital was necessary to maintain the stability and specialization of its labor base, yet the hospital's reputation as a curative institution was reliant on the quick turnover of its patient population. Stuck between its twinned objectives of therapeutic efficacy and economic self-sufficiency, the success of the hospital was predicated simultaneously on patients' absence and presence. The result of these dissonant forces was the growth of a population of a chronically ill but manageable and obedient patients whose existence sustained and justified the survival of the hospital even as it proved the failure of its foundational purpose. It is no wonder that Elizabeth Packard believed that the asylum was a machine whose primary function was the production of "incurables" (Packard 1873). In denying patients' subjectivity, refusing opportunities for reflexive self-criticism, and failing to confront the contradictions and hypocrisies of their discipline, psychiatrists cultivated an environment that was ultimately more productive of pathologies than of cures.

Discussion

The Disorderly Sensorium

This book is founded on the idea that a sensory framework offers a novel and productive means for conceptualizing the history of the asylum. By choosing to dedicate one chapter of my book to each sense, I have been able to target and explore dimensions of experience that are not readily available from other vantage points. Yet this organization has the unintended effect of eliding the dynamic interaction of the senses. The asylum was an inherently multisensory domain that engaged all of the senses simultaneously. In the everyday encounters of the asylum, sensory boundaries would have been continuously transgressed, as perceptions of numerous kinds of stimuli mixed freely.

David Howes uses the term "intersensoriality" to describe "the multi-directional interaction of the senses and of sensory ideologies, whether considered in relation to a society, an individual, or a work" (Howes 2005: 9). Intersensoriality encompasses the multifold ways in which the senses act with, upon, and against one another. The administrators of the asylum aimed at the achievement of a sensory "harmony" that would bring together all of the senses in concert to exert a holistically therapeutic effect. The sensory realms of the asylum were not intended to exist as discrete domains, but were envisioned as constitutive elements in a larger design, like instruments in an orchestra. In reality, however, sensory harmony often gave way to sensory disorder. Like the gap between theory and practice, the gap between the harmony and discord of the senses serves as a productive space for comparing the efficacy of the different sensory regimes and how their interaction functioned to alternately augment or undermine the asylum's therapeutic mission. Patients' criticism was often predicated on the juxtaposition of the different sensory orders of the asylum, which allowed them to illustrate the falsehood of the entire illusion.

Many patients pointed out the disjuncture between the asylum's idyllic appearance and the realities of confinement as informed by the other senses. Clifford Beers and Nellie Bly described the beautiful lawns of their respective asylums. Prior to her investigation, Bly had believed that the scenery of the Blackwell's Island Asylum "was such a comfort to the poor creatures confined on the Island" (Bly 1887). Once committed, she discovered that patients "are not allowed on the grass—it is only to look at." The pleasant appearance of the exterior asylum formed a thin facade over its inner realities of despair and torment and made a mockery of patients' desire for freedom. Furthermore, patients were keenly aware of the fact that the pleasant outlook of the asylum was largely targeted at visitors, not at them. Elizabeth Stone and Robert Fuller described McLean Asylum as outwardly beautiful, with a "pleasant location." Yet while administrators expended "a great deal of pains" in cultivating the "outward appearance" of the asylum, "things not seen by visiters [*sic*] are not regarded" (Stone 1842). Similarly, Ebenezer Haskell wrote that in anticipation of committees' visits to the Pennsylvania Hospital for the Insane, "everything is cleaned up in good order to deceive, so that the report will read 'in excellent condition'" (Haskell 1868: 42).

Testimonies from outsiders suggest that administrators were largely successful in this "deceit," at least in the early years of the asylum. In 1838, trustee William Lincoln praised the orderliness, neatness, and quiet of the Worcester State Hospital, stating that it bore "little resemblance to the character of an insane asylum" (Trustees Notes 1838). Visiting Worcester in 1841, Elizabeth Dorr was granted access to its grounds (though not its interiors), and wrote that "the buildings looked spacious & airy" and that the windows were designed in such a way as to "take away the unpleasant impression" of imprisonment (Dorr 1841). Both Lincoln and Dorr praised the efficacy of the asylum in disguising the reality of its function as a place for the confinement of the insane. These optical sleights-of-hand were less effective on patients. In their accounts, the lived experience of the asylum offset its aesthetic charms.

Furthermore, the gulf between the asylum's pleasant appearance and the noxious realities of the other sensory orders widened over time, becoming obvious even to casual visitors. In February 1852, trustee Samuel Gridley Howe reported that while "to the eye all was neat, orderly, and seemly" at the Worcester State Hospital, "to the smell, much was offensive, and even repulsive, especially in the strong rooms" (Trustees' Notes 1852). Similar to Walter Benjamin's "dialectical image," the smell of the strong rooms was a "dialectical odor" that "interrupt[ed] the context into which it [was] inserted," throwing the sensory harmony of the asylum into chaos (Drobnik 2005: 277). This discord represented a theater in the "moral war" between smell and vision, "with vision representing the forces of light and smell the forces of darkness" (Miller 2005: 350). While the optics of the asylum represented its therapeutic promise, its smell pointed inexorably to its physical and ideological decay. No matter how beautiful the asylum appeared, the inexorable potency of its odors would make administrators' efforts a losing battle.

Patients' accounts suggest that the visual domain of the asylum was the most easily manipulated, lending itself easily to administrators' tactics of deceit. Visual encounters with the asylum could be made from afar and for a short period, while the other sensory orders required relative proximity and the investment of time. Furthermore, administrators may have privileged sight because it was ranked first in Victorian sensory hierarchies, giving it priority as a transmitter of meaning and therapeutic device. This hierarchy of the senses was mapped onto the hierarchy of individuals who came in contact with the asylum. Those in the top tier—administrators, trustees, visitors, and upper-class patients—received greater access to its outer visual delights and were shielded from its baser elements. In contrast, attendants, housekeepers, lower-class patients, and patients in the strong rooms were largely cut off from pleasant visual stimuli and were forced to confront its repugnant interior realities. This parallel between sensory and social hierarchies was reflected in society at large, which inflected the senses with moral values and bourgeois taste, linking visual art, music, and intellectual activities to the upper classes and the pungent, tactile processes of labor to the lower classes and the enslaved. In this way, "the balance that was decreed in the use of the senses justified the logic of social cleavages" inside and outside of the asylum (Corbin 2005: 136–137).

In most cases, sensory experiences of the asylum tended not to clash with, but rather to compound one another. Many patients' accounts read as detailed sensory inventories of every kind of unpleasant stimuli, ranging from the haunting screams of fellow patients to the noxious smells of spoiled food. These stimuli were not only offensive in their own right but were also described as particularly jarring when contrasted against the familiar domestic surroundings from which patients had been removed. Patients were shocked by the experience of seeing, hearing, and smelling large groups of insane people under one roof, unrestrained by the social barriers that typically kept them apart from the rest of society. Patients were concerned both for their personal safety and for their own mental health, as they feared the contaminating influence of lunatics. As a means of reasserting a sense of order and control over their surroundings, patients staked out sensory strongholds within the asylum. Elizabeth Packard created a hygienic oasis amidst the filth of the Jacksonville Asylum by scrubbing every room and patient in her ward, while her friend Mrs. Olsen made her own body into a fortress against unwelcome sounds by stuffing her ears with cotton. Through these actions, patients actively engaged in a symbolic and physical struggle over the sensory regime of the hospital, implicitly understanding that whoever held the power to shape the sensory environment held the power to shape the bodies and minds within it.

Patients also contested the asylum's sensory regime through their written accounts, asserting their authority to create the asylum as they experienced it. One of the terms frequently invoked by patients to describe the asylum is the oxymoron "living sepulchre" (Fuller 1830). Patients likened their commitments to the asylum to being "buried alive," in the words of Lydia Denny (Denny 1862). Packard wrote that her husband "forcibly entombed me within the massive walls of the Jacksonville Asylum prison, to rise no more" (Packard 1873: 38, 121). "I am literally entombed alive by fraudulent means. The walls of my sepulcher are the walls of this asylum." Robert Fuller wrote that the asylum was "safe in the same sense, that the grave is safe," as it "shuts [patients] off from the world, and hastens [them] to death" (Fuller 1830: 27). Moses Swan described the Troy Lunatic Asylum as a "whited sepulchre . . . full of dead men's bones" (Swan 1874: 108).

There were many ways in which the asylum could "hasten" a patient toward death. Patients were allegedly burned, strangled, and drowned by abusive attendants; others died of neglect or starvation, committed suicide, or succumbed to lethal doses of chloral hydrate or to the infectious diseases that spread rapidly in crowded and unhygienic wards. Yet the "living sepulchre" described in patients' accounts is first and foremost a site of *social* death—the extinction of their identities as social beings and the slow, insidious extinction of their spirit—that stands at odds with the survival of the physical body. In invoking this term, patients may have been drawing from Percy Shelley's poem "On Love," in which he writes that "So soon as this want or power [of Love] is dead, man becomes the living sepulchre of himself, and what yet survives is the mere husk of what once he was" (Shelley 1829). Notably, Elizabeth Stone believed that the medical "treatments" she received at the McLean Asylum had rendered her incapable of love: her "body [was] dead," and her "brain [was] becoming a mineral substance . . . . the idea of love is gone from me" (Stone 1842). In patients' accounts, the "living sepulchre" of the asylum inmate who has been emptied of love and hope is paralleled by the image of the asylum as mausoleum, a repository for "dead men's bones."

THE PARADOX OF ASYLUM THERAPEUTICS

The image of the asylum conjured in patient accounts is nearly always that of a benevolent institution that has devolved into a barbaric nightmare. Patients depict the asylum as a topsy-turvy universe in which the patients are sane and the institution itself is both mad and maddening. As Clifford Beers wrote, "the treatment often meted out to insane persons is the very treatment which would deprive sane persons of their reason" (Beers 1913: 115). To use a modern medical term, the asylum was a site of iatrogenesis: the process whereby medicine *created* illness, rather than cured it. As early as 1816, the physician John Reid described English asylums as "nurseries for and manufactories of madness," in which individuals who may have only suffered from mild or temporary mental disorder were rendered mad by "barbarous and unphilosophical treatment" (Reid 1816: 723–724, 725). Despite the diffusion of moral treatment, patients' accounts throughout the nineteenth century would corroborate the notion of the maddening asylum. By 1900, the growth of asylums into "hospital palaces," populated by exponentially increasing numbers of "incurables," "seemed . . . in danger of revealing the fundamental craziness of the human mind itself" (Bynum and Shepherd 1985: 3).

Ironically, patients' invocation of iatrogenesis served the purpose of confirming, rather than challenging, the central conceit of moral treatment: that the asylum was capable of fundamentally altering its inhabitants' mood, behavior, and physical constitution. Administrators' and patients' conceptualization of the asylum was grounded in a common medical paradigm that linked body, mind, and environment and predicated health on the individual's adherence to natural laws. The point of departure between administrators and patients was positional, not ideological: a function of their differing perspective within the asylum hierarchy, rather than their differing views of the foundational principles of moral treatment. Accordingly, patients couched their criticisms of the asylum in the same medicalized language that administrators used to eulogize it. For example, administrators argued that the asylum provided a healthful refuge for the insane because it removed them from the noxious miasmas of city life. In contrast, Mrs. Olsen claimed that the environment of the Jacksonville Asylum was injurious because it provided the conditions for a different and equally pernicious kind of miasma, complaining that she was "compelled to inhale the poisonous gases from so many diseased bodies while sleeping so near each other" (Packard 1873: 326).

In making such arguments, patients chose to appropriate medical language for their own purposes, using it—as physicians did—to legitimize their claims and thereby contest physicians' monopolistic authority over the truth. Some patients appealed specifically to medical paradigms that—while considered "alternative" today—at that time posed a legitimate threat to the models espoused by asylum physicians. Elizabeth Stone invoked the tenets of phrenology to explain how the pathological environment of the asylum wreaked havoc on her vulnerable mental state. Following her release, she consulted both a "magnetized somnambulist" and several phrenologists, who diagnosed her with "distress in the back part of the head" (to which phrenology attributed the "faculties of affection"), which rendered her incapable of love and happiness (Stone 1842). All of these "experts" believed that Stone should not have been committed to an asylum. In seeking a second opinion outside of the asylum, Stone not only challenged psychiatrists' individual diagnosis but also the legitimacy of their exclusive jurisdiction over insanity. Packard posed a similar challenge when she invoked the principles of health laid down by the minister and health reformer Sylvester Graham, stating that her adherence to those principles—in defiance of institutional orders—allowed her to retain her sanity in spite of the maddening environment of the asylum.

Patients' claims served to invert the administrators' depiction of the asylum as a salutary place for unhealthy minds. The asylum's peaceful and restorative image, they claimed, formed a thin veneer over toxic practices that literally tortured, deranged, and killed patients. According to Packard, a fellow inmate who hanged herself in the asylum was "a victim to that absurd practice of the medical profession, which depends upon poisons instead of nature to cure disease" (Packard 1873: 232–233). Under these pernicious and potentially lethal conditions, patients' attempts to escape, protest, and even kill themselves could be recast as the intelligible reactions of rational beings. As Robert Fuller wrote, "it will be said that I raged during the 3 or 10 days of my imprisonment. This is true, and who could suffer as I did, and not rage?" (Fuller 1833: 20). Some physicians agreed that even sane patients could be driven to seemingly insane acts by the conditions of the asylum. Testifying in the trial of Ebenezer Haskell, Dr. S. P. Jones, who administered the male department of the Pennsylvania Hospital, described how Haskell escaped from the hospital twice by sawing through the bars of his cell, crawling through a ventilation shaft, and climbing over the wall (breaking his leg in the second attempt). Jones told the court that "I consider this no symptom of insanity. [The hospital] is not a pleasant place for some men" (Haskell 1868: 9).

Patients knew that their claims to sanity were not only necessary to legitimize their claims but also served to further tarnish the reputation of the asylum and the legitimacy of psychiatry. They may have recognized, as psychiatrists certainly did, that the emergent discipline of psychiatry stood on shaky ground as a medical "science" that claimed the ability to diagnose patients on the basis of protean and subjective standards of sanity. The lack of objective diagnostic criteria in psychiatry was particularly damning when contrasted against the increasingly visible and tangible pathologies uncovered by other fields of medicine through the use of autopsy and microscopy. Physicians in those fields could point confidently to the seat of physical disease in the body. In contrast, Lydia Denny wrote that "[i]t is an easy thing for Dr. Tyler to say that it is his opinion that I am insane, but is Dr. Tyler infallible?" (Denny 1862). As long as psychiatrists failed to localize insanity in the brain or other parts of the body, that question would continue to hang over the discipline.

Nellie Bly's work of investigative journalism, during which she feigned symptoms of insanity in order to gain access to the Blackwell's Island Asylum, struck a particularly damaging blow. Bly wrote that once her diagnosis was secured, "the more sanely I talked and acted the crazier I was thought to be" (Bly 1887). In fact, her fellow patients proved more perceptive than her physicians in detecting Bly's sanity. According to Bly, many of these patients were sane themselves, but had ended up in the asylum through some combination of poverty, sickness, and inability to speak fluent English. Similarly destructive to the legitimacy of psychiatry were the accounts of Lydia Denny and Elizabeth Packard, who blamed their commitments on patriarchal laws that allowed their respective husbands to confine them without cause; both women were ultimately vindicated in the courts. Like Bly, Denny, and Packard questioned their physicians' ability to distinguish the sane from the insane, with Denny suggesting that her physician's "opinion" of her insanity was based on a conspiratorial consensus with her husband rather than proper diagnostic methods. "No injured wife can obtain a divorce from an unfaithful husband," she wrote, "if he chooses to say she is insane" (Denny 1842: 13).

Thus, at a time when psychiatry was struggling to secure its authority over insanity through appeals to scientific objectivity, patients pointed out the flaws and inconsistencies in psychiatric reasoning and offered their own experiences as proof of their physicians' failures. In making such claims, patients challenged psychiatrists' perceptions in much the same way that psychiatrists challenged theirs, claiming that *they,* the purportedly insane, were more effective arbiters of sanity than their purportedly "infallible" physicians. Packard targeted the foundations of the discipline at its most vulnerable points, challenging Dr. McFarland to "test your transcendental machinery and power to make out a case of insanity, as so occult a nature, that no being in the universe has ever had any evidence of its existence in any plane whatever, either physical, mental, moral or spiritual" (Packard 1873: 123).

The menace that Packard's authority—as a female patient who had been declared sane by the courts—posed to the overwhelmingly male class of psychiatrists is suggested by their hostile and sexist reactions to her. In their 1872 annual meeting, members of the AMSAII discussed the passage of so-called "Packard Laws" in Iowa that put checks on asylum superintendents' power to censor and withhold patient letters from their intended recipients. The psychiatrists disapproved of the law, which they viewed as an imposition on their jurisdiction as superintendents and a threat to the hierarchy of the asylum. According to this law, "all letters may be sent, not directly to friends, but to a committee (lawyer, physician, and lady of the state), who have the power to read them and judge of the propriety of sending them to their destination" ("Proceedings" 1872: 255). The members proceeded to disparage the authority of this "lady" through projected associations with Packard, insanity, and the women's rights movement (ibid.).

Dr. Kirkbride: Is the lady reliable?

Dr. Ranney: I do not know personally. She is a lady of high character and influence in the State at large, a lady of culture and refinement, I believe. But what course will be pursued by this committee, I have no means of determining.

Dr. Walker: Has this lady on the committee had any communication with Mrs. Packard?

Dr. Raney: I do not know of my own knowledge; but I think there are but few persons in the more populous portions of the State who have not had communication with [Packard]. She has been industriously circulating her publications, and I presume there are very few persons in the state who have no information of them.

Dr. Walker: Has that lady ever been insane?

Dr. Ranney: I think not, sir.

Dr. Workman: Is she a woman's rights woman? (Laughter.)

While the authority of Packard's, Denny's, and Bly's accounts hinged on their claims to sanity, other patients acknowledged that they had once suffered from mental disorder while maintaining their claims of ill-treatment. While the asylum could drive a sane person mad, they believed, it could also make a mad person worse. Elizabeth Stone wrote that the McLean Asylum "is to a weak excited persons as a grog-shop to an intemperate man, or a house of ill-fame, to a licentious person; they can be completely ruined" (Stone 1842). Administrators were quick to disregard the complaints of inmates as the ravings of madmen. In contrast, Hunt entreated his readers to "think not that a mad man raves," asserting that even an insane person could tell the truth. Finding the trustees unwilling to entertain his complaints of abuse, Hunt stated, "Whether you will believe it or not it is nevertheless true" (Hunt 1851: 11).

What were the conditions that were capable of turning a sane mind mad? Most patient accounts describe the abuse committed by attendants, whose authority was enforced by intimidation and violence. Some of the "treatments" patients received—such as forced feeding and "hydrotherapy" that forced distressed patients underwater—were virtually indistinguishable from torture. Medical treatment was at best ineffective and at worst actively harmful; in many cases, patients believed it was not "medicine" at all. Packard believed that "all the 'medical treatment' [patients] get here, is that of locks and keys" (Packard 1873: 234). While many patients complained of abuse, they were just as likely to complain that attendants ignored them. Under conditions of overcrowding and insufficient staffing, individualized attention—the backbone of moral treatment—was virtually impossible. As Beers wrote, "for one year no further attention was paid to me than to see that I had three meals a day, the requisite number of baths, and a sufficient amount of exercise" (Beers 1913: 35). Yet as Beers and many other patients attest, sometimes even these bare necessities were lacking.

In addition to these overt complaints, patients described the more insidious afflictions of confinement, including feelings of boredom, homesickness, loneliness, despair, and shame. While many of the hardships of the asylum may be attributed at least partly to the vagaries of the asylum in practice— such as improper administration, insufficient staffing and resources, and the general decline of therapeutic optimism — these afflictions were endemic to the asylum as it was originated. Asylum treatises consistently endorsed the separation and isolation of patients from their families and communities as a necessary precondition for recovery. Anticipating the distress that this might cause, administrators worked to make the asylum a welcoming environment and provide opportunities for recreation and entertainment. Their intention was to encourage patients' "emplacement" within the asylum, in order to achieve a harmonious "interrelationship of mind-body-environment" (Howes 2005: 7). Instead, the asylum largely functioned as a mechanism of "displacement," making patients feel "homeless [and] disconnected from [their] physical and social environments" (ibid.). Denny wrote that her separation from her friends and family filled her with "unutterable anguish," and described her life at the McLean Asylum as "a daily and deadly humiliation" (Denny 1862). Upon his admission to McLean in 1832, Robert Fuller "felt myself shut out from the world," and "shuddered to think of my family deprived of their natural protector" (Fuller 1833: 15). Despite administrators' efforts to ameliorate the stigmatic aspects of the asylum, patients suffered from the knowledge that they were inmates in an institution. Bly wrote that "excepting the most violent cases, [patients] are conscious that they are confined in an asylum. The only desire that never dies is the one for release, for home" (Bly 1887).

Despite these grievances, patients did not contest the legitimacy of the asylum as an idea. Moses Swan wrote that "I am not altogether opposed to these institutions, for there are insane persons who have no homes," and hoped that asylums might be reformed in order to "become what they were originally designed for" (Swan 1874: 91, 63). Elizabeth Stone had "no dispute but what there should be an institution as an Insane Assylum [*sic*]"; rather, she protested the fact that its power been invested in "the hands of a few individuals, over a distressed class of beings, a money-making system, at the expense of happiness" (Stone 1842). Notably, Elizabeth Packard believed that "kind, humane, Christian treatment" *was* available: at the Worcester State Hospital, where one of her fellow patients had been formerly committed under the superintendence of Dr. Woodward. Upon her removal from Worcester to Jacksonville, however, this patient "received such a shock, followed by such a feeling of degradation and shame, that it has become impossible for her to rally and recover her lost self-respect" (Packard 1873: 272).

In their efforts to make their suffering legible to their readers, many patients invoked what they believed was the most appropriate analog: slavery. The "peculiar institution" served as a useful shorthand for brutality, persecution, inhumanity, and wrongfully circumscribed freedom. By drawing such comparisons, patients were able to mobilize the rhetoric of the well-established genre of anti-slavery discourse and thereby appeal to the same sympathies. Both Denny and Packard wrote (practically verbatim) that "the insane have no rights that the sane are bound to respect," echoing the infamous words of Chief Justice Roger Taney in the ruling of *Scott v. Sanford* in 1857 (Denny 1862). While the allusion in Denny's statement is implied, Packard makes it explicit, adding: "no, not even so much as the slaves are" (Packard 1873: 110). Similarly, Stone wrote that she would happily trade places with a slave rather than remain an inmate of the asylum (Stone 1842). These words were carefully calculated to tap into the same vein of outrage and animate the same reformatory zeal as abolitionism.

Ironically, similar rhetoric and sentiments, targeting the public conscience and sense of decency, had been used decades earlier to galvanize the asylum movement. To give credence to her crusade, Dix had written vividly of lunatics "confined . . . in *cages, closets, cellars, stalls, pens! Chained, naked, beaten with rods,* and *lashed* into obedience!" (Dix 1843). Both the asylum movement and its later reformatory campaigns hinged on the public's visceral reaction to scenes of abuse and degradation. In perfecting this rhetorical device, patients' accounts drew liberally from the genre of slave narratives and thereby invoked the same twinned claims of personal vindication and social justice. As Fuller wrote, "When one has been falsely accused, imprisoned, and persecuted nearly unto death, it is both his right and duty to make such an exposition of the whole affair as will tend to prevent its recurrence" (Fuller 1833: 9).

It is worth noting that all of the aforementioned patients' accounts were written by white Northerners, a fact that simultaneously deflates and enhances the legitimacy of their moral crusade. From the point of view of their (largely white, educated) intended audiences, the imprisonment and persecution of a white person may have seemed to amplify their sense of outrage. The dissemination of photographs of light-skinned enslaved children—"as white, as intelligent, as docile, as most of our own children"—as a method for inciting outrage among audiences who were, apparently, not outraged enough by the horrors of black slavery, suggests that white people valued white freedom more highly and were more likely to react to the mistreatment of a white person (Mitchell 2014).

From a more modern vantage point, patients authors' lack of familiarity with slavery somewhat undermines the basis for their comparison. These writers "experienced" slavery only as it was refracted through news accounts and anti-slavery tracts, which they eagerly emulated for their own devices. In contrast, many millions of people in the United States at the time *did* possess intimate knowledge of slavery; however, their representation in asylum narratives is lacking. In the Southern states, black people—whether slave or free—were largely barred from state hospitals, while northern asylums kept black patients in segregated wards. At Worcester, administrators' conviction that "Africans" "ought not to mingle with the other female patients" justified the confinement of black patients to separate quarters (Trustees' Notes 1833). The narrative of a black patient, who could testify from the "nexus of blackness and madness," would make an invaluable addition to the genre of patient accounts (Gilman 1985). Without this testimony, however, the experiences of these patients—as well as many other marginalized groups in the asylum—can be glimpsed only indirectly, and through the narratives of patients who had the resources, education, and opportunity to make their voices heard. Their stories provide a crucial, though inevitably biased, window into the asylum experience.

THE FAILURE OF EMPATHY

For much of the history of the asylum, administrators framed the problems they faced in primarily logistical terms, portraying the administration of the asylum as a conglomerate of Sisyphean tasks. The ever-expanding population of patients, the budgetary restraints placed on the maintenance and expansion of the asylum, and the poorly trained and overworked employees speak to the incongruence between the lofty mission of the asylum, and the resources it was given to accomplish its objectives. It is easy to imagine how one superintendent, tasked with the care and treatment of as many as 3,000 patients, could fail to address the complaints of every individual. Yet patients' accounts did not focus on benign acts of oversight on the part of overburdened employees, but targeted the failure of administrators to register their complaints as valid. The problem was not that the administrators could not hear patients' complaints or lacked the resources to address them, but that they refused to listen. In the words of Isaac Hunt, they "shut their ears, closed their eyes and barricaded their hearts, sympathy and human feeling against my plaintive story—a truthful recital of my wrongs, sufferings, and deprivations" (Hunt 1851: 13).

This failure on the part of administrators was partly a function of the effect of positionality on sensory perception. Administrators did not perceive the same stimuli as patients did. Because sensory experience "is not just something one sees or hears about; it is something one *lives*" (Howes 2005: 3), simply being present in the asylum environment did not provide administrators with the *experience* of commitment and its correspondent emotions and insights. While they may have heard the screams of patients and smelled the rank odor of the strong rooms, they didn't *feel* them in the way that patients did. This positional anesthesia was not only an unfortunate byproduct of administrators' place in the asylum hierarchy but also an instrumental and defining function of it. Administrators had ample incentive *not* to register their patients' perceptions of the asylum as pathological and abusive, as doing so would threaten both their personal authority and the validity of the asylum model and the discipline of psychiatry. While many of these administrators may have raised the same concerns about hygiene, neglect, and disrepair, they didn't regard them with the same sense of outrage and urgency as patients did. To administrators, these patients were simply being insane or hysterical and couldn't be trusted to impart an accurate judgment of their own circumstances.

While administrators acknowledged that *patients* experienced the asylum differently according to their backgrounds and levels of education, they did not acknowledge the role that *their own* identities—as white men of an elite and educated class—played in shaping their perceptions of the asylum and the way it was administered. Gerald Grob has suggested that in the early decades of the Worcester State Hospital, a shared class identity provided an accessible platform upon which patients and superintendents could meet, leveling the power differential between patient and physician (Grob 1966). The efficacy of moral treatment was predicated on the meeting of physician and patient on these relatively equal terms. During these years, Woodward visited every patient in the hospital daily and often invited patients to dine with his family. In contrast, as patients and physicians became increasingly separated by barriers of class, race, and nativity, superintendents began to regard patients as inferiors and treated them with a correspondent degree of disdain and distance. The belief that immigrants and paupers were considered less amenable to treatment became a self-fulfilling prophecy in the second half of the nineteenth century. Grob attributes the decline in the therapeutic function of the asylum to the failure of moral treatment to bridge the divide between physicians and patients of disparate backgrounds.

Yet the relationship between physician and patient was also an inherently *unequal* one within the context of the asylum, even if they were of similar standing in society. The efficacy of treatment depended on this "natural" power inequity, as it enabled the physician to assume the position of authority that was necessary to guide the patient back to health. This dynamic may have lent itself more readily to the treatment of female patients, whose subordinate position to men was naturalized by society (Hewitt 2015; Bynum and Shepherd 1985; Tomes 1984). Male superintendents easily stepped into the paternalistic role played by women's fathers and husbands and mobilized it as a therapeutic measure. While Elizabeth Packard sharply criticized the law that made her a "legal nonentity" whose "personal liberty depended entirely upon the will or wishes of my husband," she was not a proponent of the women's rights movement and believed that "in reality there is no higher office a woman can fill than that of maternity" (Packard 1873: 195). In fact, her criticisms of Dr. McFarland partly targeted his failure to protect her, which she regarded as a renunciation of his manhood: "Woman was made *to be* protected by man." Despite psychiatrists' representation of her, Packard sought foremost to *enforce* the patriarchy by shielding women against the abuse of men's power and reminding men of their natural duty as benevolent protectors. She was not interested in dismantling patriarchy itself.

Similarly, patients did not seek to repudiate the asylum model itself, but rather protested its perversion in the hands of corrupt, greedy, and sadistic individuals. While intended as a panacea for the evils of modernity, patients believed that the asylum had been infected by the soulless cupidity of capitalism, pointing to the dirty compromises that administrators made between therapeutics and profit. In the words of Clifford Beers, a "spirit of economy and commercialism pervaded the entire institution" (Beers 1913: 21). Patients believed that administrators profited from the unremunerated labor of patients and thus had an incentive to accept the admissions of people who were not insane and delay the release of those who had recovered. Swan believed that sane patients at the Troy Lunatic Asylum were "kept as slave[s] to do drudgery for the benefit of the stockholders of the institution at the expense of tax payers in the county of Rensselaer" (Swan 1874: 118). Packard quoted an attendant who informed her that "the Doctor [McFarland] keeps sane people here from choice, knowing that the unrequited labor he gets out of them he can turn to his aggrandizement—in his report of the finances of the institution" (Packard 1873: 2014). Whether or not these conspiratorial theories were true, patients' statements express a keen awareness of the conflict between their roles as both patients and institutionalized laborers.

Under the constraints of this exploitive system, some patients entertained the idea that their captors were downright evil. Hunt claimed that his complaints were suppressed because the superintendent of the Maine State Hospital, Dr. Bates, "was afraid that I should expose his villainy . . . that then he would not be able to swell and parade upon his portico, like Nebuchadnezzar upon his palace walls" (Hunt 1851: 17). Packard "believe[d] that it was the Doctor's purpose to make a maniac of me, by the skillful use of asylum tortures" (Packard 1873: 113). Swan aimed his ire at his attendants, writing: "The Devil is the father of the Cain family and the father of lies, and almost all the attendants of lunatic asylums are graduates or pupils in that family" (Swan 1874: 86). Patients who rejected their diagnoses eagerly redirected the charge of insanity toward their captors. Swan states that "I thought my attendants were lunatics" (ibid.: 49). Packard informed Dr. McFarland that "you have exhibited more evidence of insanity than I have seen on any person since I entered this institution" (Packard 1873: 123). In making these statements, patients claimed their authority over the truth, using the label of insanity to refute administrators' legitimacy as truth-tellers in the same way that administrators used it to deny theirs.

Conclusion
The Afterlife of the Asylum

The narrative of the curative lunatic hospital devolving into a snakepit runs through the history of asylums, mirroring the turn from optimism to pessimism over the course of the nineteenth century (Cherry 1989; Gamwell and Tomes 1985; Grob 1966). At the Worcester State Hospital, evidence for the inversion from therapeutic to pathological can be found in every sphere of its sensory assemblage. Access to pleasant views of nature and surrounding gardens was destroyed by the encroachment of urbanization and the development of the hospital grounds. The ideal of a quiet, peaceful environment gave way to the cacophony of the overcrowded asylum. The initial monumentality and solidity of the hospital building was degraded by neglect and disrepair so that the same architectural features and materials that had indexed progress for one generation became associated with backwardness and neglect. The hospital's pure atmosphere came to be sullied by the same problems of sanitation and hygiene from which it was intended to provide a refuge, and the healthful diet it purported to provide was steadily replaced by poor substitutes that literally starved patients of necessary nutrients.

All of these factors were cited justifiably as claims against the asylum during the mid-twentieth-century deinstitutionalization movement. However, as critics of deinstitutionalization have argued, the outright repudiation of the asylum obscures its promise and early successes, resulting in a kind of "amnesia" whereby the discipline has lost sight of the valuable insights and knowledge of its predecessors (Etzioni 1975: 12). As asylum medicine evolved into psychiatry, the conceptualization and treatment of insanity shifted from environmental to biomedical paradigms, with the result that the asylum model has been replaced by one predicated largely on psychoactive medication and outpatient treatment. Even in the relatively small number of in-patient facilities that remain in the United States, the physical structure of the psychiatric hospital is no longer considered a therapeutic modality in itself: it is a place of cure, rather than a curative place.

Since the mid-twentieth century, anthropological approaches to insane asylums and other total institutions have been shaped by the work of Michel Foucault, Erving Goffman, and other theorists working within a social control model (Bynum and Shepherd 1985; Bivins and Pickstone 2007; Luhrman 2001; Sedgwick 1982). However, this model has been challenged by anthropologists, archaeologists, and historians who point to the many individual contingencies that it obscures or omits, and who demonstrate the value of a fine-grained approach that takes into account the material and spatial dimensions of power and the inflections of individual agency and experience (Luhrmann 2001; Mills 2000; Murat 2014; Porter 2002; Reiss 2008; Piddock 2007). Asylum medicine was predicated on a sensory approach to the treatment of insanity: specifically, upon the creation of a curative environment intended to maximize patients' exposure to restorative sensory stimuli (Piddock 2007; Yanni 2007). In the preceding pages, my aim has been to access those stimuli as they were refracted through the ideological and physical structures of the asylum, for the purpose of reconstructing the sensorial assemblage of the Worcester State Hospital. In doing so, I have sought to define how experiences of confinement are formed in the interface between individual historical agents and the institutional environment, through the spaces, materials, and activities of everyday life.

With the deinstitutionalization movement, the sensory order of the asylum has collapsed, leading to the dispersal of the experiences that it once organized across space and time. Many of the former patients of Massachusetts state hospitals ended up on the streets or in temporary shelters for the mentally ill established by the Department of Mental Health, such as the one visited by anthropologist Robert Desjarlais during his fieldwork in the early 1990s. In contrast to the ordered and at times mind-numbingly predictable sensory regime of the asylum, Desjarlais describes the "sensorium of the street" as "a corporeal existence in which a person's senses and the ability to make sense soon became dulled in response to excessive and brutal demands on those senses" (Desjarlais 2005: 372). The actions of people in a temporary shelter in Boston represent strategies to reclaim the kind of regularity and control that the asylum once offered by "set[ting] up routines in order to mediate the distractions" of everyday life and trying to "settle in" to the shelter in a way that renders their surroundings comfortable and familiar (ibid.: 374–375). Patients' descriptions of the remedial effects of routine on their illness recalls Clifford Beers's statement that "the even-going routine of institutional life . . . affords the indispensable quieting effect—provided that routine is well ordered, and not defeated by annoyances by ignorant or indifferent doctors or attendants" (Beers 1913: 33).

Having "settled in" to the shelter, residents often resisted the efforts of staff members to "move [them] along." In a remarkable inversion of the traditional asylum narrative—in which patients strive to escape or secure their release while administrators conspire to keep them confined—residents of this "no-man's limbo for the displaced" express their desire to put down "roots" in the shelter. Whether out of "fond[ness]" for the shelter or fear of the world beyond it, they preferred this relative degree of stability and permanence over the transitory and unpredictable existence on the streets (Desjarlais 2005). The accounts of Desjarlais's informants at the shelter are corroborated by other former inmates of state hospitals who found themselves displaced by the processes of deinstitutionalization. For all of the imperfections of the state hospital system—and there were many—patients did succeed in carving out a place for themselves within the alienating and distressing environment of the asylum. In the words of one former patient of the Craig Dunain Asylum in Scotland, "That awful place was home" (Parr 2003)—a statement that speaks to the "ambiguous legacy" of the asylum as both a prison and a shelter (Morrissey and Goldman 1980).

While many state hospitals have been shuttered completely, those that continue to operate do so on a much-reduced scale relative to the mid-twentieth century. As the Worcester Recovery Center and Hospital, the former Worcester State Hospital holds the capacity for only 320 patients, a smaller number than it held in 1840. The imposing Kirkbride building, which had been vacated at the time of the devastating fire in 1991, was finally demolished in 2008 and replaced with a far smaller facility organized on the pavilion plan, with separate wings that radiate from a central hub. Relative to the nineteenth-century hospital, the rate of turnover is high; patients receive treatment for days or weeks rather than months or years. In contrast to the nineteenth-century asylum, which was designed to accommodate patients with varying degrees and types of insanity, the residents of the twenty-first-century hospital tend to suffer from more severe illnesses; those with "minor" illnesses are treated on an outpatient basis or, in many cases, do not receive treatment at all. Security is rigidly enforced; patients do not wander across the grounds or journey several miles to neighboring Shrewsbury to work on the asylum farm as they did in the nineteenth and early twentieth centuries, but are rather restricted to a small courtyard enclosed by a high wire fence.

Like the nineteenth-century asylum, the design of the twenty-first-century hospital reflects its uses and priorities. It is a place of transition, rather than residence; a hospital, rather than a home. The environment is not vested with agency but rather represents a neutral and sterilized backdrop for medical treatment. Accordingly, the organization and functioning of the twenty-first-century hospital owes little to the legacy of its predecessor, the asylum. For all their grievances against the asylum, patients may have been dismayed to learn that the asylum model has been almost entirely repudiated. Elizabeth Packard believed that "all the good which inheres in this institutions and officers is just as precious as if not mixed with the alloy; therefore, in destroying the alloy, great care should be used not to tarnish or destroy the fine gold within it" (Packard 1873: 400). She identified the Worcester State Hospital as one institution where the doctrine of moral treatment was upheld. Similarly, while Clifford Beers wrote extensively of the abuses he suffered at the first asylum to which he was committed, he attributed his ultimate recovery to the treatment he subsequently received at another hospital, where the "environment [was] more nearly in tune with my ill-tuned mind" (Beers 1913: 34).

For all of their grievances, patients did not reject the underlying logic of the asylum as a curative environment and bemoaned the waste of its potential. While confined to the Troy Lunatic Asylum, Moses Swan recalled a "beautiful garden, inclosed with a gate, a vineyard forming a shady walk, thorny hedge, and trees bearing fruit" (Swan 1874). Despite visiting the asylum several times after his release, he failed to locate the garden. Most likely, it had been sacrificed to the meet the asylum's increasing demand for residential or agricultural space. To Swan, the disappearance of the garden represented the asylum's fall from grace; he asked, "Who hath sinned?" Administrators' optimistic confidence in the power of the environment to cure insanity may appear fatally naive in retrospect—yet I would argue that it is worthwhile to study this early and seemingly innocent era in the history of asylums. While Swan's garden may reflect an Edenic vision of the asylum that never truly existed in reality, historical studies have suggested that there are valuable lessons to be salvaged from the ruins of the asylum.

Recently, mental health advocates have fought to reassert the role of the environment in shaping subjectivities within the psychiatric hospital. In 2015, an unprecedented law passed in Massachusetts granted the right to "daily access to fresh air and the outdoors" to the residents of in-patient psychiatric facilities (Grohol 2015). With this "Fresh Air Act," the state wrote into law a principle that was embodied in the earliest asylum designs, when Massachusetts first extended the humanistic, optimistic—and as yet unfulfilled—promise to its mentally ill citizens: that the state would not only alleviate their suffering, but provide the means for a cure.

Bibliography

1830. "Resolve for erecting a lunatic hospital, 10 March 1830." In *Reports and Other Documents Relating to the State Lunatic Hospital at Worcester, Mass.* Boston: Dutton and Wentworth, Printers to the State.

1832. "Communication from Commissioners and Trustees, 6 December 1832." In *Reports and Other Documents Relating to the State Lunatic Hospital at Worcester, Mass.* Boston: Dutton and Wentworth, Printers to the State.

1833–1924. Trustees' Notes. State Hospital at Worcester Records. American Antiquarian Society, Worcester, Massachusetts.

1833–1940. *Annual Report of the Trustees of the State Lunatic Hospital at Worcester.* Boston: Dutton & Wentworth, State Publishers.

1833. "Bill for Building Trask's Room." State Lunatic Hospital Filings. Massachusetts State Archives, Boston, Massachusetts.

1833. *System of Regulations for the State Lunatic Hospital, Worcester, Mass.* Worcester: Printed by S. H. Colton and Co.

1833. "Trask Caught." *Boston Post*, 8 May, 2.

1835. "Specifications of the Additions to be Made to the Present Building at the State Lunatic Hospital at Worcester." State Lunatic Hospital Filings. Massachusetts State Archives, Boston, Massachusetts.

1836. "Scene at an Insane Hospital." *American Magazine* III (1).

1837. *Hymns for the Hospital Chapel, Worcester.* Worcester: Mirick and Bartlett.

1838. "Thanksgiving at the Lunatic Asylum." *New-Bedford Mercury* XXII (25).

1838. "Thanksgiving at the State Lunatic Hospital, at Worcester." *Connecticut Courant* LXXIV (3856): 1.

1845. "Notices of Books: *Journal of Prison Discipline and Philanthropy.*" *American Journal of Insanity* 1 (4): 381.

1846. "Case of Mental Excitement Allayed by Music." *The American Journal of Insanity* 3 (2): 149–150.

1849. "View of Worcester from the Insane Hospital." In *Some Historic Houses of Worcester.* Printed for Worcester Bank and Trust Company, 27. Boston, MA:

Copied, arranged and printed by direction of Walton Advertising & Printing Company.

1851. "Report on the Construction of Hospitals for the Insane, Made by the Standing Committee of the Association of Medical Superintendents of American Institutions for the Insane, at its meeting in Philadelphia, May 21, 1851." *American Journal of Insanity* 8 (1): 79–80.

1861. "Insanity in Massachusetts." *American Journal of Insanity* 18 (1): 94–95.

1865. "On Separate Asylums for Curables and Incurables." *American Journal of Insanity* 22 (2): 246–252.

1870. "Report of a Committee of the Council Appointed to Investigate Certain Charges Against the Trustees and Officers of the Northampton Lunatic Hospital." Boston: Wright & Potter, State Printers.

1872. "Proceedings of the Association." *American Journal of Insanity* 29 (2): 137–263.

1876. "Proceedings of the Association." *American Journal of Insanity* 32 (3): 161–323.

1876. "The Treatment of Insanity in America." *American Journal of Insanity* 32 (3): 440–447.

1877. "An Important Public Structure Completed: Description of the Edifice." Newspaper clipping. Worcester Historical Museum, Worcester, Mass.

1878. "Proceedings of the Association." *American Journal of Insanity* 35 (1): 74–181.

1878. "Report of the Proceedings of the New England Psychological Society." *American Journal of Insanity* 34 (4): 531–534.

1878. "Illness of Colonel Washburn." Newspaper clipping. Washburn Correspondence, 1878-1886. American Antiquarian Society, Worcester, Massachusetts.

1879. "Proceedings of the Association." *American Journal of Insanity* 36 (2): 139–223.

1884. "Proceedings of the Association." *American Journal of Insanity* 41 (1): 40–100.

1886. "Notes: Uniforming Attendants." *American Journal of Insanity* 43 (1): 127–128.

1887. "Notes: The Electric Light in Asylums." *American Journal of Insanity* 43 (3): 391–392.

1888. "Mental Affections and Aural Disease." *American Journal of Insanity* 44 (3): 410.

1888. "Proceedings of the Association." *American Journal of Insanity* 45 (1): 65–162.

1889. "Proceedings of the Association." *American Journal of Insanity* 46 (2): 224–281.

1890. "Proceedings of the Association." *American Journal of Insanity* 47 (2): 166–240.

1891. "Proceedings of the association." *American Journal of Insanity* 48 (1): 71–104.

1895. "The Favorable Modification of Undesirable Symptoms in the Incurable Insane." *American Journal of Insanity* 51 (4): 449–458.

1902. "Nurses in Rebellion: Strike and Lockout at State Insane Hospital." *Boston Herald,* 28 August. Newspaper clipping. Worcester Historical Museum, Worcester, Massachusetts.

1902. "Put Out Bag and Baggage!: Hospital Nurses Try to Take What They Want and Find It Doesn't Work." *Worcester Telegram,* 29 August. Newspaper clipping. Worcester Historical Museum, Worcester, Massachusetts.

1902. Untitled newspaper clipping. *Worcester Sunday Herald.* Worcester Historical Museum, Worcester, Massachusetts.

1913. "Great waste of food at hospital." Newspaper clipping, November 7. Worcester Historical Museum, Worcester, Massachusetts.

1922. *Annual Report of the Memorial Hospital.* Worcester: Press of Charles Hamilton.

1935. "Facility survey, Hooper Turret." State Hospital Facility Surveys. Massachusetts State Archives, Boston, Massachusetts.

1946. "Pre-frontal Lobotomy." *The Messenger* 20 (4).

1983. "Tour of Worcester State Hospital." Worcester Historical Museum, Worcester, Massachusetts.

2009. "Highway of Commerce: The Blackstone Canal." Worcester Historical Museum. http://www.worcesterhistory.org/ex_blackstone1.html.

2019. Entry for Hope Cemetery. Massachusetts Cultural Resource Information System (MACRIS). http://mhc-macris.net/Details.aspx?MhcId=WOR.B.

Adams Nervine Asylum. 1880. *Proposed Rules and Regulations of the Adams Nervine Asylum: to Be Considered at a Meeting of the Managers to be Held February 28, 1880.* Boston: s. n.

Allen, Nathan. 1880. *Supervision of Lunatic Hospitals.* Boston: Tolman & White, Printers.

Alberti, Benjamin. 2018. "Art, Craft, and the Ontology of Archaeological Things." *Interdisciplinary Science Reviews* 43 (3–4): 280–294.

Alleridge, Patricia. 1985. "Bedlam: Fact or Fantasy?" In *The Anatomy of Madness: Essays in the History of Psychiatry,* edited by W. F. Bynum and M. S. Shepherd, 17–32. London: Tavistock Publications.

Allmond, Gillian. 2015. "Light and Darkness in an Edwardian Institution for the Insane Poor: Illuminating the Material Practices of the Asylum Age." *International Journal of Historical Archaeology* 20 (1–22).

Andrén, Anders. 1998. *Between Artifacts and Texts: Historical Archaeology in Global Perspective.* New York: Plenum Press.

Andrews, Jonathan. 1998. "Case Notes, Case Histories, and the Patient's Experience of Insanity at Gartnavel Royal Asylum, Glasgow, in the Nineteenth Century." *Social History of Medicine* 11 (2): 255–281.

Ashmore, W. and A. B. Knapp, eds. 1999. *Archaeology of Landscape: Contemporary Perspectives.* Oxford: Blackwell.

Bancroft, J. P. 1889. "The Bearing of Hospital Adjustments Upon the Efficiency of Remedial and Meliorating Treatment in Mental Diseases." *American Journal of Insanity* 45 (3): 374–386.

Barstow, Ann. 1994. *Witchcraze: A New History of the European Witch Hunts.* San Francisco and London: Pandora.

Baugher, Sherene. 2010. "Landscapes of Power: Middle-Class and Lower-Class Power Dynamics in a New York Charitable Institution." *International Journal of Historical Archaeology* 14: 475–497.

Bauman, Zygmunt. 1993. "The Sweet Scent of Decomposition." In *Forget Baudrillard?* edited by Chris Rojek and Bryan S. Turner, 24-28. New York: Routledge.

Beers, Clifford W. 1913. *A Mind That Found Itself: An Autobiography.* London: Longmans, Green, & Co.

Beisaw, A. M. and J. G. Gibb. 2009. *The Archaeology of Institutional Life.* Tuscaloosa: University of Alabama Press.

Bell, Luther V. 1845. "Modern Improvements in the Construction, Ventilation, and Warming of Buildings for the Insane, with a Design for the 'Butler Hospital for the Insane' at Providence, RI." *American Journal of Insanity* 2 (1): 13–33.

Bell, Luther V. 1850. "On the Coercive Administration of Food to the Insane." *American Journal of Insanity* 6 (3): 223–234.

Bell, Vaughn. 2011. "A Whiff of Madness." Mind Hacks. https://mindhacks.com /2011/09/11/a-whiff-of-madness/.

Beveridge, Allan. 1997. "Voices of the Mad: Patients' Letters from the Royal Edinburgh Asylum, 1873-1908." *Psychological Medicine* 27 (4): 899–908.

Biehl, Jao. 2013. *Vita: Life in a Zone of Social Abandonment.* Berkeley: University of California Press.

Bivins, R. E. and J. V. Pickstone. 2007. *Medicine, Madness, and Social History: Essays in Honour of Roy Porter.* Basingstoke: Palgrave Macmillan.

Black, J. R. 1873. *The Ten Laws of Health: or, How Disease is Produced and Can be Prevented.* J. B. Lippincott & Co., Philadelphia.

Blackwood R. D. 1872. "The Maid of Sker." *Blackwood's Edinburgh Magazine* DCLXXV (CXI).

Blanchard, Mary E. to Benjamin Seaver. 23 April 1854. Letters to Benjamin Seaver, 1824-1854. Massachusetts Historical Society, Boston, Mass.

Blumer, G. Alder. 1892. "Music in Its Relation to the Mind." *American Journal of Insanity* 48 (3): 350–365.

Bly, Nellie. 1887. *Ten Days in a Mad-House.* Ian L. Munro, New York.

Boerhaave, Herman. 1724. *Boerhaave's Aphorisms: Concerning the Knowledge and Cure of Diseases.* London: Printed for William and John Innys.

Brian, K. M. 2012. "'Occasionally Heard to be Answering Voices': Aural Culture and the Ritual of Psychiatric Audition, 1877-1911." *History of Psychiatry* 23 (3): 305–317.

Browne, W. A. F. 1837. *What Asylums Were, Are, and Ought to Be.* Edinburgh: Adam and Charles Black.

Browne, W. A. F. 1875. "Artificial Alimentation." *American Journal of Insanity* 31 (3): 305–335.

Buchanan, J. M. "Insanity in the Colored Race." *American Journal of Insanity* 43 (2): 278–280.

Bucknill J. C. 1876. "Notes on Asylums for the Insane in America." *American Journal of Insanity* 33 (2): 137–160.

Burley, David V. 1989. "Function, Meaning, and Context: Ambiguities in Ceramic Use by the *Hivernant* Metis of the Northwestern Plains." *Historical Archaeology* 23 (1): 97–106.

Burton, Robert. 1621. *The Anatomy of Melancholy: What It Is, With all the Kindes, Cases, Symptomes, Prognostickes, and Several Causes of It.* Oxford: John Lichfield and James Short.

Bushman R. L. 1993. *The Refinement of America.* New York: Vintage Books.

Buttolph, H. A. 1847. "Modern Asylums, and Their Adaptation to the Treatment of the Insane." *American Journal of Insanity* 3 (4): 364–378.

Bynum, W. F. and M. S. Shepherd. 1985. *The Anatomy of Madness: Essays in the History of Psychiatry.* London: Tavistock Publications.

Bynum, W. F. and R. Porter, eds. 1993. *Medicine and the Five Senses.* Cambridge, UK: University Press.

Callaway, Enoch. 2007. *Asylum: A Mid-Century Madhouse and its Lessons about Our Mentally Ill Today.* Connecticut and London: Praeger.

Camal, Jerome. 2019. "An Anthropology of Sound? Schultze's Sonic Meditations, from Helmholz to Webern on Mars." *Sound Studies* 5 (2): 194–197.

Camp, Stacey Lynn. 2016. "Landscapes of Japanese American Internment." *Historical Archaeology* 50 (1): 169–186.

Carpenter, A. N. 1885. *A Few Hints on Landscape Architecture, as Applied to the Home, the Farm, Parks, Cemeteries, Public Institutions, Fair and Assembly Grounds.* Gallesburg, Ill.: [s.n.].

Casella Eleanor C. 2001. "To Watch or Restrain: Female Convict Prisons in 19th-Century Tasmania." *International Journal of Historical Archaeology* 5 (1): 45–72.

Casella, Eleanor C. 2009. "On the Enigma of Incarceration: Philosophical Approaches to Confinement in the Modern Era." In *The Archaeology of Institutional Life,* edited by A. M. Beisaw and J. G. Gibb, 17–32. Tuscaloosa: University of Alabama Press.

Chapin John B. 1892. "Suggestions for Improved Plans for Treatment of Recent and Recoverable Cases of Insanity." *American Journal of Insanity* 49 (2): 184–191.

Chapin, John B. 1883. "Public Complaints Against Asylums for the Insane, and the Commitment of the Insane." *American Journal of Insanity* 40 (1): 33–50.

Chapin, John B. 1889. "Address Delivered at the 43rd Annual Meeting of the AMSAII, Newport, Rhode Island, June 18, 1889." *American Journal of Insanity* 46 (91): 1–21.

Charland, Louis C. 2007. "Benevolent Theory: Moral Treatment at the York Retreat." *History of Psychiatry* 18: 61–80.

Cherry, Charles L. 1989. *A Quiet Haven: Quakers, Moral Treatment, and Asylum Reform.* London and Toronto: Associated University Press.

Cheyne, George. 1642. *The Natural Method of Cureing the Diseases of the Body, and the Disorders of the Mind Depending on the Body.* London: Printed for Geo. Strahan and John and Paul Knapton.

Classen, Constance. 1997. "Foundations for an Anthropology of the Senses." *International Social Science Journal* 49 (153): 409–410.

Cocks, Catherine. 2001. *Doing the Town: The Rise of Urban Tourism in the United States, 1850-1915.* Berkeley: University of California Press.

Coleborne, Catharine and Dolly MacKinnon, eds. 2003. *"Madness" in Australia: Histories, Heritage and the Asylum.* St. Lucia: University of Queensland Press.

Collins, Ellen to Pliny Earle. 25 July 1874. Pliny Earle Papers. American Antiquarian Society, Worcester, Massachusetts.

The Commissioners of Hope Cemetery. 1865. "Annual Report of the Commissioners of Hope Cemetery." In *City Document No. 20: Inaugural Address of Hon. James B. Blake, Mayor of the City of Worcester, with the Annual Reports of the Several City Officers.* Worcester: Tyler & Seagrave.

The Commissioners of Hope Cemetery. 1872. "Annual Report of the Commissioners of Hope Cemetery." In *City Document No. 26: Inaugural Address of Hon. George F. Verry, Mayor, Jan. 1, 1872, with the Annual Reports ...* Worcester: Printed by Edward R. Fiske, Crompton's Block.

The Commissioners. 1832. "Report of the Commissioners Appointed to Superintend the Erection of a Lunatic Hospital at Worcester, January 4, 1832." In *Reports and Other Documents Relating to the State Lunatic Hospital at Worcester, Mass.* Boston: Dutton & Wentworth.

Conolly, John. 1847. *The Construction and Government of Lunatic Asylums and Hospitals for the Insane.* London: Dawsons of Pall Mall.

Corbin, Alain. 1986. *The Foul and the Fragrant: Odor and the French Social Imagination.* Cambridge, MA: Harvard University Press.

Corbin, Alain. 2005. "Charting the Cultural History of the Senses." In *Empire of the Senses: The Sensual Culture Reader,* edited by David Howes, 128–137. Oxford and New York: Berg.

Coventry, C. B. 1846. "Physiology of the Brain." *American Journal of Insanity* 3: 198–200.

Cox, Joseph Mason. 1811. *Practical Observations on Insanity.* Philadelphia: Published by Thomas Dobson, at the Stone House, No. 41, South Second Street, Fry and Kammerer, Printers.

Crichton, Alexander. 1798. *An Inquiry into the Nature and Origin of Mental Derangement.* London: T. Cadell.

Davies, Kerry. 2007. "'A Small Corner That's for Myself': Space, Place, and Patients' Experience of Mental Health Care, 1948-98." In *Madness, Architecture, and the Built Environment: Psychiatric Spaces in Historical Context,* edited by Leslie Topp, James E. Moran, and Jonathan Andrews, 304–314. London and New York: Routledge.

Davis, G. 2008. *"The Cruel Madness of Love": Sex, Syphilis and Psychiatry in Scotland, 1880-1930.* Amsterdam: Rodopi.

Dawson, Joanna. 2003. "Pottery from the Royal Edinburgh Asylum." Thesis, University of Glasgow.

Dawson, P., et al. 2007. "Simulating the Behaviour of Light inside Arctic Dwellings: Implications for Assessing the Role of Vision in Task Performance." *World Archaeology* 39 (1): 17–35.

Day, Jo, ed. 2013. *Making Senses of the Past: Toward a Sensory Archaeology.* Carbondale and Edwardsville: Center for Archaeological Investigations, Southern Illinois University Carbondale, Occasional Paper No. 40. Southern Illinois University Press.

De Cunzo, Lu Ann. 1995. "Reform, Respite, Ritual: An Archaeology of Institutions: The Magdalen Society of Philadelphia, 1800-1850." *Historical Archaeology* 29 (3): i–168.

Deetz, James. 1996. *In Small Things Forgotten: An Archaeology of Early American Life.* New York: Random House.

Delle, James A. 1998. *The Archaeology of Social Space: Analyzing Coffee Plantations in Jamaica's Blue Mountains.* New York: Plenum Press.

Denny, Lydia B. 1862. *Statement of Mrs. Lydia B. Denny, Wife of Reuben S. Denny, of Boston: In Regard to her Alleged Insanity.* Boston: [s.n.].

Desjarlais, Robert. 2005. "Movement, Stillness: On the Sensory World of a Shelter for the 'Homeless Mentally Ill.'" In *Empire of the Senses: The Sensual Culture Reader,* edited by David Howes, 369–379. Oxford and New York: Berg.

Deutsch, Albert. 1946. *The Mentally Ill in America: A History of their Care and Treatment from Colonial Times.* New York: Columbia University Press.

Deutsch, Albert. 1948. *The Shame of the States.* New York: Harcourt, Brace and Company.

Digby, Anne. 1985. "Moral Treatment at the Retreat, 1796-1846." In *The Anatomy of Madness: Essays in the History of Psychiatry,* edited by W. F. Bynum & M. S. Shepherd, 52–63. London: Tavistock Publications.

Dix, Dorothea Lynde. 1843. *Memorial to the State of Massachusetts.* Boston: Munroe & Francis.

Dodd, James. 2017. *Phenomenology, Architecture, and the Built World: Exercises in Philosophical Anthropology.* Boston: Brill.

Dorr, Elizabeth. 1841. Elizabeth Dorr Diaries, 1835-1859. Massachusetts Historical Society, Boston, Massachusetts.

Douglas, Mary. 1966. *Purity and Danger: An Analysis of the Concepts of Pollution and Taboo.* London: Routledge.

Drobnik, Jim. 2005. "Volatile Effects: Olfactory Dimensions of Art and Architecture." In *Empire of the Senses: The Sensual Culture Reader,* edited by David Howes, 265–280. Oxford and New York: Berg.

Durkheim, Emile. 1951. *Suicide: A Study in Sociology.* New York: Simon and Schuster.

Dwyer, Ellen. 1987. *Homes for the Mad: Life Inside Two Nineteenth-Century Asylums.* New Brunswick, NJ and London: Rutgers University Press.

Earle, Pliny to Clinton D. Miner. 18 April 1878. Pliny Earle Papers. American Antiquarian Society, Worcester, Massachusetts.

Earle, Pliny. 1844. "A Leaf from and for the *Annals of Insanity.*" Pliny Earle Papers. American Antiquarian Society, Worcester, Massachusetts.

Earle, Pliny. 1845. "Historical and Descriptive Account of the Bloomingdale Asylum for the Insane." *American Journal of Insanity* 2 (1): 1–12.

Earle, Pliny. 1847. "Cases of Paralysis Peculiar to the Insane: The Paralysic Generale of the French, from the *American Journal of the Medical Sciences* XIII, April." Pliny Earle Papers. American Antiquarian Society, Worcester, Massachusetts.

Earle, Pliny. 1849. "Cases of Partio-General Paralysis, from the *American Journal of the Medical Sciences,* Jan. 1849." Pliny Earle Papers. American Antiquarian Society, Worcester, Massachusetts.

Earle, Pliny. 1877. "The Curability of Insanity." *American Journal of Insanity* 33 (4): 483–533.

Earle, Pliny. 1879. *A Glance at Insanity and the Management of the Insane in the American States.* Boston: Franklin Press.

Earle, Pliny. 1887. "The Curability of Insanity: Study First Written in 1876." In *The Curability of Insanity: A Series of Studies* by Pliny Earle. Philadelphia: Lippincott, 1887.

Earle, Pliny. 1898. *Memoirs of Pliny Earle.* Boston: Damrell & Upham.

Earle, Pliny. 1845. "The Poetry of Insanity." *American Journal of Insanity* 1 (3): 193–224.

Eaton, Leonard K. *New England Hospitals, 1790-1833.* Ann Arbor: The University of Michigan Press, 1957.

Edginton B. 2007. "A Space for Moral Management: The York Retreat's Influence on Asylum Design." In *Madness, Architecture, and the Built Environment: Psychiatric Spaces in Historical Context,* edited by Leslie Topp, James E. Moran, and Jonathan Andrews, 85–104. London and New York: Routledge.

El-Hai, J. 2005. *The Lobotomist: A Maverick Medical Genius and His Tragic Quest to Rid the World of Mental Illness.* Hoboken, NJ: John Wiley & Sons, Inc.

Ellis, Charles M. 1866. *Argument of C. M. Ellis, Esq.: Before the Committee of the City Government, on the Memorial of Oliver Frost, Touching the Management of the Lunatic Hospital, November 10, 1865.* Boston: Nation Press, J. M. Usher.

Ellis, W. C. 1838. *A Treatise on the Nature, Symptoms, Causes, and Treatment of Insanity, With Practical Observations on Lunatic Asylums.* London: Samuel Holdsworth, Amen Corner.

Epperson, T. W. 1990. "Race and the Disciplines of the Plantation." *Historical Archaeology* 24 (4): 29–36.

Erickson, Pamela I. 2003. "Medical Anthropology and Global Health." *Medical Anthropology Quarterly* 17: 3–4.

Esquirol, Etienne. 1845. *Mental Maladies: A Treatise on Insanity.* Translated from the French, with additions, by E. K. Hunt. Philadelphia: Lea and Blanchard.

Etzioni, A. 1975. "Deinstitutionalization: A Public Policy Fashion." *Human Behavior* 4 (9): 12–13.

Evans W. F. 1872. *Mental Medicine: A Theoretical and Practical Treatise on Medical Psychology.* Boston: Carter & Pettee.

Everts, Orpheus. 1881. "The American System of Public Provision for the Insane, and Despotism in Lunatic Asylums." *American Journal of Insanity* 38 (2): 113–139.

Falret, Henri. 1854. "On the Construction and Organization of Establishments for the Insane." *American Journal of Insanity* 10 (3): 218–262.

Feld, Steven, and Donald Brenneis. 2004. "Doing Anthropology in Sound." *American Ethnologist* 31 (4): 461–474.

Fennelly, K. 2014. "Out of Sound, Out of Mind: Noise Control in Early 19th-Century Lunatic Asylums in England and Ireland." *World Archaeology* 46 (3): 416–430.

Fitts, R. K. (1996). "The Landscapes of Northern Bondage." *Historical Archaeology* 30 (2): 54–73.

Forbes, Winslow. 1868. *Light: Its Influence on Life and Health.* New York: Moorhead, Simpson, & Bond.

Foucault, Michel. 1977. *Madness and Civilization: A History of Insanity in the Age of Reason.* New York: New American Library.

Fowler, O. S. 1856. *Sexual Diseases: Their Causes, Prevention, and Cure, on Physiological Principles.* New York: Fowler and Wells.

Franklin, B. 2002. "Hospital - Heritage - Home: Reconstructing the Nineteenth-Century Lunatic Asylum." *Housing, Theory, and Society* 19: 170–184.

Fraser, K. 1998. "The Photographic Insane." *Cinémas (Montréal)* 9 (1): 139–149.

Frost, Henry Pinkney. 1917. *Boston State Hospital: Dorchester Centre, Mass.* Reprinted from The Institutional Care of the Insane in the United States and Canada II.

Fuller, Robert. 1833. *An Account of the Imprisonment and Sufferings of Robert Fuller, of Cambridge.* Boston: Printed for the author.

Gamwell, Lynn and Nancy Tomes. 1984. *Madness in America: Cultural and Medical Perceptions of Mental Illness Before 1914.* Binghamton, NY: State University of New York.

Gardner, E. C. 1874. *Homes and How to Make Them.* Boston: James R. Osgood and Company.

Gaston, William. 1877. *Argument of Hon. William Gaston in Relation to the New Lunatic Hospital at Danvers, Mass.* Boston: Albert J. Wright, State Printer.

Gilman, S. L. 1985. "Difference and Pathology: Stereotypes of Sexuality, Race, and Madness." Ithaca: Cornell University Press.

Godding W. W. 1890. "Aspects and Outlook on Insanity in America." *American Journal of Insanity* 47 (1): 1–17.

Godding, W. W. 1877. "Taunton." *American Journal of Insanity* 33 (4): 541–543.

Godding, W. W. 1884. "Progress in Provision for the Insane, 1844-1884." *American Journal of Insanity* 41 (2): 129–150.

Goffman, Erving. 1961. *Asylums: Essays on the Social Situation of Mental Patients and Other Inmates.* Garden City, NY: Anchor Books.

Golden, Janet. 1982. "Custody and Control: The Rhode Island State Hospital for Mental Diseases, 1870-1970." *Rhode Island History* 41 (4): 113–125.

Goldman, Howard H. 1980. "Changing Organizational Boundaries: A Socio-Ecological Perspective." In *The Enduring Asylum: Cycles of Institutional Reform at Worcester State Hospital* by Joseph P. Morrissey, Howard H. Goldman, Lorraine V. Klerman, and associates, 127–142. New York: Grune & Stratton.

Gollaher, David. 1995. *Voice for the Mad: The Life of Dorothea Dix.* New York: The Free Press.

Godden, Geoffrey A. 1999. *Godden's Guide to Ironstone China and Granite Wares.* Antique Collectors' Club Ltd., Woodbridge, Suffolk.

Gosden, Christopher. 1994. *Social Being and Time.* Oxford: Blackwell.

Gray, John P. 1871. *Insanity: Its Dependence on Physical Disease.* Utica, NY: Roberts, Book and Job Printer.

Gray, John P. 1874. "Pathology of Insanity." *American Journal of Insanity* 31 (1): 1–29.

Griesinger, W. 1866. "The Mental Operations in Health and Disease." *American Journal of Insanity* 22 (3): 308–333.

Grob, Gerald N. 1966. *The State and the Mentally Ill: A History of the Worcester State Hospital in Massachusetts, 1830-1920.* Chapel Hill: University of North Carolina Press.

Grohol, John M. 2015. "Massachusetts Psychiatric Patients Get Right to Fresh Air." *Psych Central.* 11 March. https://psychcentral.com/blog/massachusetts-psychiatric -patients-get-right-to-fresh-air/.

Hacking, Ian. 1985. "Making Up People." In *Reconstructing Individualism,* edited by T. L. Heller, M. Sosna, and D. E. Wellbery. Stanford: Stanford University Press.

Haddad, John R. 2007. "Imagined journeys to distant Cathay: Constructing China with ceramics, 1780-1920." *Winterthur Porfolio* 41 (1): 53–80.

Hall, Martin and Stephen W. Silliman, eds. 2006. *Historical Archaeology.* Malden, MA: Blackwell.

Hamilakis, Yannis. 2014. *Archaeology and the Senses: Human Experience, Memory and Affect.* Cambridge: Cambridge University Press.

Hamlett, J. 2013. "Comfort in Small Things? Clothing, Control, and Agency in County Lunatic Asylums in 19th- and Early 20th-Century England. *Journal of Victorian Culture* 18 (1): 93–113.

Haskell, Ebenezer. 1869. *The Trial of Ebenezer Haskell, in Lunacy, and His Acquittal Before Judge Brewster, in November, 1868.* Philadelphia: Published by the Author.

Heidegger, Martin, ed. 1971. *Poetry, Language, Thought.* New York: Harper Colophon.

Helmreich, Stefan. 2007. "An Anthropologist Underwater: Immersive Soundscapes, Submarine Cyborgs, and Transductive Ethnography." *American Ethnologist* 34 (4): 621–641.

Hewitt, J. 2015. "Women Working 'Amidst the Mad': Domesticity as Psychiatric Treatment in 19th-Century Paris." *French Historical Studies* 38 (1): 105–137.

Hickman, Clare. 2009. "Cheerful Prospects and Tranquil Restoration: The Visual Experience of Landscape as part of the Therapeutic Regime of the British Asylum, 1800-60." *History of Psychiatry* 20 (4): 425–441.

Hill, Elizabeth R. 1881. *False Imprisonment of Elizabeth R. Hill by Rev. Gabriel H. De Bevoise, and the Selectmen of North Brookfield, Mass. Jan. 5, 1878, and Incidents Resulting Therefrom to Feb. 15, 1881.* Entered according to Act of Congress, on the 24th of May, in the year 1881, by Elizabeth R. Hill, in the Office of the Librarian of Congress, at Washington.

Houston, Robert A. 2000. *Madness and Society in Eighteenth-Century Scotland.* Oxford: Oxford University Press.

Howell, Michael and Peter Ford. 1992. *The True History of the Elephant Man.* London: Penguin Books.

Howes, David, ed. 2005. *Empire of the Senses: The Sensual Culture Reader.* Oxford and New York: Berg.

Hrdlička, Ales. 1899. "Art and Literature in the Mentally Abnormal." *American Journal of Insanity* 55 (3): 371–404.

Hubert, Jane. 2000. *Madness, Disability, and Social Exclusion: The Archaeology and Anthropology of "Difference."* London and New York: Routledge.

Hughes, C. H. 1874. "Psychical or Physical." *American Journal of Insanity* 31 (1): 30–49.

Hunt, Isaac. 1851. *Astounding Disclosures! Three Years in a Mad House: By A Victim: Written By Himself.* Entered according to an act of Congress, in the year 1851, by Isaac H. Hunt, in the Clerk's Office of the District Court of Massachusetts.

Hurd, Henry. 1883. "Summary: Ducking: A Refutation." *American Journal of Insanity* 39 (4): 506–507.

Husserl, Edmund. 1960. *Cartesian Meditations: An Introduction to Phenomenology.* The Hague: M. Nijhoff.

Hutchinson, Francis. 1718. *An Historical Essay Concerning Witchcraft.* London: Printed for R. Knaplock, at the Bishop's Head, and D. Midwinter, at the Three Crowns in St. Paul's Church-yard.

Inspectors of Prisons. 1848. *Reports of the Inspectors of Prisons, of the County of Suffolk, on the Jail, House of Reformation, House of Industry, Boston Lunatic Hospital, and House of Correction. December 1848.* Boston: J. H. Eastburn, City Printer.

Jackson, D. D. 2011. "Scents of place: The displacement of a First Nations community in Canada." *American Anthropologist* 113 (4): 606–618.

Jarvis, Edward to Almira Jarvis. 1860. Edward Jarvis Letters. American Antiquarian Society, Worcester, Massachusetts.

Jarvis, Edward. 1841. *Insanity and Insane Asylums.* Louisville, KY: Prentice and Weissinger.

Jarvis, Edward. 1855. *Insanity and Idiocy in Massachusetts: Report of the Commission on Lunacy, 1855.* Cambridge: Harvard University Press.

Jarvis, Edward. 1865. "Curability of the Insane." *American Journal of Insanity* 22: 255.

Jennings, Chris. 2016. *Paradise Now: The Story of American Utopianism.* New York: Random House.

Johnson, A. B. 1856. *The Physiology of the Senses; Or, How and What We See, Hear, Taste, Feel and Smell.* New York: Derby and Jackson, Publishers.

Johnson, Matthew. 2012. "Phenomenological Approaches in Landscape Archaeology." *Annual Review of Anthropology* 41: 269–284.

Joyce, Rosemary. 2005. "Archaeology of the Body." *Annual Review of Anthropology* 34: 139–158.

Kane, Michael D. 2015. "Historic Clock Tower of Worcester State Hospital Gets New Life." *MassLive,* 10 December. www.masslive.com/news/worcester/2015/12/historic_clocktower_of_worcest.html.

Kellogg, M. G. 1874. *The Hygienic Family Physician: A Complete Guide for the Preservation of Health, and the Treatment of the Sick Without Medicine, Comprising Also a Valuable Pamphlet on Diet.* Battle Creek, Michigan: Published at the Office of the Health Reformer.

Kim, D. Y. 2016. "Psychiatric Deinstitutionalization and Prison Population Growth." *Criminal Justice Policy Review* 27 (1): 3–21.

Kirkbride, Thomas S. 1854. *On the Construction, Organization, and General Arrangements of Hospitals for the Insane.* Philadelphia: [s.n.].

Kleinman, Arthur, Veena Das, and Margaret Lock, eds. 1997. *Social Suffering.* Berkeley: University of California Press.

Kleinman, Arthur. 2001. "Why Psychiatry and Cultural Anthropology Still Need Each Other." *Psychiatry* 64 (1): 14–16.

Kromm, Jane. 2007. "Site and Vantage: Sculptural Decoration and Spatial Experience in Early Modern Dutch Asylums." In *Madness, Architecture, and the Built Environment: Psychiatric Spaces in Historical Context,* edited by Leslie Topp, James E. Moran, and Jonathan Andrews, 19–39. London and New York: Routledge.

Leatherman, Tom and Alan H. Goodman. 2011. "Critical Biocultural Approaches in Medical Anthropology." In *Companion to Medical Anthropology,* edited by Merrill Singer and Pamela I. Erickson, 29–47. Oxford, UK: Wiley-Blackwell.

Lee J. E. 1847. "Escapes from Lunatic Asylums. *American Journal of Insanity* 3 (3): 202–211.

Léger, Daniel. 2008. "Scurvy: Reemergence of Nutritional Deficiencies" *Canadian Family Physician/Medecin De Famille Canadien* 54 (10): 1403–1406.

Leidesdorf, Maximilian. 1865. "Pathologico-Anatomical Manifestations of Insanity." *American Journal of Insanity* 22 (2): 147–190.

Leone, Mark P. 2005. *The Archaeology of Liberty in an American Capital: Excavations in Annapolis.* Berkeley: University of California Press.

Leone, Mark P. and Constance A. Crosby. 1987. "Middle-Range Theory in Historical Archaeology." In *Consumer Choice in Historical Archaeology,* edited by Suzanne Spencer-Wood, 397–410. New York: Plenum Press.

Leone, Mark P. and Parker B. Potter. 1999. *Historical Archaeologies of Capitalism.* New York: Kluwer Academic/Plenum Publishers.

Little, Nina Fletcher. 1972. *Early Years of the McLean Hospital: Recorded in the Journal of George William Folsom, Apothecary at the Asylum in Charlestown.* Boston, MA: The Francis A. Countway Library of Medicine.

Locke, John. 1853. *An Essay Concerning Human Understanding and a Treatise on the Conduct of the Understanding.* Philadelphia: Troutman & Hayes.

Luhrmann, T. M. 2001. *Of Two Minds: An Anthropologist Looks at American Psychiatry.* New York: Vintage Books.

MacKinnon, Dolly. 2003. "'Hearing Madness': The Soundscape of the Asylum." In *"Madness" in Australia: Histories, Heritage, and the Asylum,* edited by Catharine Coleborne and Dolly MacKinnon, 73–82. St. Lucia: University of Queensland Press.

Mange, Paul to Rockwood Hoar. 16 December 1902. Rockwood Hoar Papers. Massachusetts Historical Society, Boston, Massachusetts.

Markowitz, F. E. 2006. "Psychiatric Hospital Capacity, Homelessness, and Crime Arrest Rates." *Criminology* 44 (1): 45–72.

Marsh, James L. 1988. *Post-Cartesian Meditations: An Essay in Dialectical Phenomenology.* New York: Fordham University Press.

Martin, S. A. 2007. "Between Kraepelin and Freud: The Integrative Psychiatry of August Hoch." *History of Psychiatry* 18 (71): 275–299.

Mather, Cotton. 1692. *The Wonders of the Invisible World: Being an Account of the Tryals of Several Witches Lately Executed in New England.* London: John Russell Smith.

Mayne, Alan. 2008. "On the Edges of History: Reflections on Historical Archaeology." *The American Historical Review* 113 (1): 93–118.

McAtackney, L. and R. Palmer. 2016. "Colonial Institutions: Uses, Subversions, and Material Afterlives." *International Journal of Historical Archaeology* 20: 471–476.

Mill, John Stuart. 1836. "Civilization." *London and Westminster Review*: 130–131.

Miller, George L. 1991. "A revised set of CC index values for classification and economic scaling of English ceramics from 1787 to 1880." *Historical Archaeology* 25 (1): 1–25.

Miller, William Ian. 2005. "Darwin's Disgust." In *Empire of the Senses: The Sensual Culture Reader,* edited by David Howes, 335–354. Oxford and New York: Berg.

Mills, J. 2000. "The Mad and the Past: Retrospective Diagnosis, Post-Coloniality, Discourse Analysis, and the Asylum Archive." *Journal of Medical Humanities* 21 (3): 141–158.

Miner, Clinton D. to Pliny Earle. 16 September 1878. Pliny Earle Papers. American Antiquarian Society, Worcester, Massachusetts.

Mitchell, Juliet. 2000. *Mad Men and Medusas: Reclaiming Hysteria.* New York: Basic Books.

Mitchell, Mary Niall. 2014. "The young white faces of slavery." *The New York Times,* 30 January. https://opinionator.blogs.nytimes.com/2014/01/30/the-young-white-faces-of-slavery/.

Mitchell, S. Weir. 1877. *Fat and Blood: and How to Make Them.* Philadelphia: J. B. Lippincott & Co.

Morison, Alexander. 1837–1848. *A Collection of Original Drawings by Roshard, A Johnson, Gow etc. made to illustrate the works of Sir Alexander Morison on Mental Diseases.* Collection of Sir Alexander Morison. Royal College of Physicians of Edinburgh, Edinburgh.

Morris, O. W. 1851. "An Inquiry Whether Deaf Mutes are More Subject to Insanity than the Blind." *American Journal of Insanity* VIII (1): 18.

Morrissey, Joseph P., Howard H. Goldman, Lorraine V. Klerman, and associates. 1980. *The Enduring Asylum: Cycles of Institutional Reform at Worcester State Hospital.* New York: Grune & Stratton.

Morrissey, Joseph P., Howard H. Goldman, and Lorraine V. Klerman. 1980. "Approaches to the Study of Institutional Reform." In *The Enduring Asylum: Cycles of Institutional Reform at Worcester State Hospital,* by Joseph P. Morrissey, Howard H. Goldman, Lorraine V. Klerman, and Associates, 1–16. New York: Grune & Stratton.

Morrison, Hazel. 2016. "Constructing Patient Stories: 'Dynamic' Case Notes and Clinical Encounters at Glasgow's Gartnavel Mental Hospital, 1921-32." *Medical History* 60: 67–86.

Morrissey, Joseph P. and Howard H. Goldman. 1980. "The Ambiguous Legacy, 1856-1968." In *The Enduring Asylum: Cycles of Institutional Reform at Worcester State*

Hospital, by Joseph P. Morrissey, Howard H. Goldman, Lorraine V. Klerman, and associates, 45–95. New York: Grune & Stratton.

Murat, Laure. 2014. *The Man Who Thought He Was Napoleon: Toward a Political History of Madness.* Chicago and London: University of Chicago Press.

Myerson, David J. 1980. "Deinstitutionalization and Decentralization, 1969-1977." In *The Enduring Asylum: Cycles of Institutional Reform at Worcester State Hospital* by Joseph P. Morrissey, Howard H. Goldman, Lorraine V. Klerman, and associates, 97–123. New York: Grune & Stratton.

Nightingale, Florence. 1860. *Notes on Nursing: What It Is, and What It Is Not.* New York: D. Appleton and Company.

Nutt, Charles. 1919. *History of Worcester and Its People, Vol. III.* New York: Lewis Historical Publishing Company.

Nylander, Richard C. 2016. "Framing the Interior: The Entrepreneurial Career of John Doggett." *Publications of the Colonial Society of Massachusetts, Vol. LXXXVIII: Boston Furniture 1700-1900,* edited by Brock Jobe and Gerald W. R. Ward. Boston: Colonial Society of Massachusetts.

Olsen, Bjornar. 2010. *In Defense of Things: Archaeology and the Ontology of Objects.* Lantham, MD: AltaMira Press.

Owen, Robert Dale. 1849. *Hints on Public Architecture.* New York: Putnam.

Packard, E. P. W. 1873. *Modern Persecution: Or Insane Asylums Unveiled as Demonstrated by the Report of the Investigating Committee of the Legislature of Illinois.* Hartford: Case, Lockwood & Brainard, Printers.

Palmer, O. H. 1878. "Suicide Not Evidence of Insanity." *American Journal of Insanity* 34 (4): 425–461.

Parigot, J. 1863. "General Mental Therapeutics." *American Journal of Insanity* 19 (4): 381–405.

Parkman, G. 1817. *Management of Lunatics with Illustrations of Insanity.* Boston: Printed by John Eliot.

Parr, H. 2003. "'That Awful Place Was Home': Reflections on the Contested Meanings of Craig Dunain Asylum." *Scottish Geographical Journal* 119 (4): 341–354.

Payne, Christopher. 2009. *Asylum: Inside the Closed World of State Mental Hospitals.* Cambridge, MA: Massachusetts Institute of Technology.

Philo, Chris. 2007. "Scaling the Asylum: Three Geographies of the Inverness District Lunatic Asylum (Craig Dunain)." In *Madness, Architecture, and the Built Environment: Psychiatric Spaces in Historical Context,* edited by Leslie Topp, James E. Moran, and Jonathan Andrews, 105–130. London and New York: Routledge.

Picker, J. M. 2003. *Victorian Soundscapes.* Oxford: Oxford University Press.

Piddock, Susan. 2007. *A Space of their Own.* New York: Springer.

Pinel, Philippe. 1962. *A Treatise on Insanity.* New York: Hafner Pub. Co.

Porter, Roy. 2002. *Madness: A Brief History.* Oxford: Oxford University Press.

Porter, Roy. 1985. "The Patient's View: Doing Medical History from Below." *Theory and Society* 14 (2): 175–198.

Ray Isaac. 1863. *Mental Hygiene.* Boston: Ticknor and Fields.

Ray, Isaac. 1846. "Observations on the Principal Hospitals for the Insane, in Great Britain, France, and Germany." *American Journal of Insanity* 2 (4): 290–378.

Ray, Isaac. 1852. "The Popular Feeling Towards Hospitals for the Insane." *American Journal of Insanity* 9 (1): 36–65.

Ray, Isaac. 1863. *Mental Hygiene.* Boston: Ticknor & Fields.

Ray, Isaac. 1870. "Address Delivered at the Laying of the Corner Stone of the State Hospital for the Insane, at Danville, Penn., August 26, 1869." *American Journal of Insanity* 26 (4): 426–449.

Reaume, Geoffrey. 2000. *Remembrance of Patients Past: Patient Life in the Toronto Hospital for the Insane, 1870-1940.* Oxford: Oxford University Press.

Reid, A. P. to Pliny Earle. 25 January 1879. Pliny Earle Papers. American Antiquarian Society, Worcester, Massachusetts.

Reid, John. 1816. "Essays on Insanity, Hypochondriasis, and Other Nervous Affections." London: Longman et al.

Reiss, B. 2008. *Theaters of Madness: Insane Asylums and Nineteenth-Century American Culture.* Chicago and London: University of Chicago Press.

Rothman, David J. 2002. *The Discovery of the Asylum: Social Order and Disorder in the New Public.* New York: Aldine de Gruyter.

Rush, Benjamin. 1812. *Medical Inquiries and Observations Upon the Diseases of the Mind.* Philadelphia: Kimber & Richardson.

Rush, Benjamin. 1872. *An Account of the Causes and Indications of Longevity, and of the State of Body and Mind in Old Age, with Observations on its Diseases, and their Remedies.* New York: Poole & MacClauchlan, Printers.

Sacks, Oliver. 2009. "Introduction." In *Asylum: Inside the Closed World of State Mental Hospitals,* by Christopher Payne. Cambridge, MA: Massachusetts Institute of Technology.

Sanborn, Arthur M. to Rockwood Hoar. 9 December 1898. Rockwood Hoar Papers. Massachusetts Historical Society, Boston, Massachusetts.

Sanborn, F. B. 1877. *The Hospital Palace at Danvers: Argument of F. B. Sanborn Before the Committee to Investigate the Cost of the Danvers Hospital.* [S.l.]: [s.n.]. Massachusetts Historical Society, Boston, Massachusetts.

Scheper-Hughes, Nancy. 1989. "Three Propositions for a Critically Applied Medical Anthropology." *Papers: Kroeber Anthropological Society* 69: 62–71.

Scot, Reginald. 1584. *The Discoverie of Witchcraft.* London: William Brome.

Scott, J. C. 1990. *Domination and the Arts of Resistance: Hidden Transcripts.* New Haven: Yale University Press.

Scull, Andrew. 1979. *Museums of Madness: The Social Organization of Insanity in Nineteenth-Century England.* New York: St. Martin's Press.

Scull, Andrew. 1981. *Madhouses, Mad-Doctors, and Madmen: The Social History of Psychiatry in the Victorian Era.* Philadelphia, PA: University of Pennsylvania Press.

Sedgwick, Peter. 1982. *Psycho Politics: Laing, Foucault, Goffman, Szasz, and the Future of Mass Psychiatry.* New York: Harper & Row.

Shackel, Paul A. 1993. *Personal Discipline and Material Culture.* Knoxville: University of Tennessee Press.

Shanks, Michael. 2012. *The Archaeological Imagination.* Left Coast Press, Walnut Creek.

Shelley, Percy. 1829. "On Love." In *The Keepsake for 1829,* edited by Frederic Mansel Reynolds, 47–49. London: Hurst, Chance, & Co.

Singer, Merrill and Pamela I. Erickson, eds. 2011. *Companion to Medical Anthropology.* Oxford, UK: Wiley-Blackwell.

Skålevåg, S. A. 2002. "Constructing Curative Instruments: Psychiatric Architecture in Norway, 1820-1920." *History of Psychiatry* 13 (49): 51–68.

Skey, Frederic Carpenter. 1867. *Hysteria.* London: Longmans, Green, Reader, & Dyer.

Smith, Leonard. 2008. "'Your Very Thankful Inmate': Discovering the Patients of an Early County Lunatic Asylum." *Social History of Medicine* 21 (2): 237–252.

Smith, Leonard. 2014. *Insanity, Race and Colonialism: Managing Mental Disorder in the Post-Emancipation British Caribbean, 1838-1914.* London and New York: Palgrave Macmillan.

Smith, Mark M. 2006. *How Race is Made: Slavery, Segregation, and the Senses.* Chicago: University of Chicago Press.

Sorensen, Tim Flohr. 2015. "Book Review: *Archaeology and the Senses* by Yannis Hamilakis." *Current Anthropology* 56 (6): 928–931.

Southwick, Albert B. 2012. "The Clock Tower Controversy." *Worcester Telegram and Gazette,* 3 May. www.telegram.com/article/20120503/COLUMN21/105039865.

Spencer-Wood, Suzanne M. 2010. "Feminist Theoretical Perspectives on the Archaeology of Poverty: Gendering Institutional Lifeways in the Northeastern United States from the Eighteenth Century through the Nineteenth Century." *Historical Archaeology* 44 (4): 110–135.

Spencer-Wood, Suzanne M. and Sherene Baugher. 2001. "Introduction and Historical Context of the Archaeology of Institutions of Reform. Part I: Asylums." In *Special Issue: The Archaeology of Institutions of Reform, Part I: Asylums,* edited by Suzanne M. Spencer-Wood and Sherene Baugher. *International Journal of Historical Archaeology* 5 (1): 3–18.

Spurzheim, J. G. 1833. *Observations on the Deranged Manifestations of the Mind, Or Insanity.* Boston: Marsh, Capen & Lyon.

State Lunatic Hospital Filings, 1830-1838, Commonwealth of Massachusetts State Archives, Boston, Massachusetts.

Stearns, H. P. 1884. "Progress in the Treatment of the Insane." *American Journal of Insanity* 41 (1): 22–39.

Stolz, John. 1872. *Treatise on the Five Senses.* Chicago: Evening Post Printing House.

Stone, Elizabeth T. 1842. *A Sketch of the Life of Elizabeth T Stone and of Her Persecutions with an Appendix of Her Treatment and Sufferings While in the Charlestown McLean Asylum, Where She Was Confined Under the Pretense of Insanity.* S.l.: Printed for the author.

Strong, Jamin to Pliny Earle. 6 December 1888. Pliny Earle Papers. American Antiquarian Society, Worcester, Massachusetts.

Surface-Evans, S. L. 2016. "A Landscape of Assimilation and Resistance: The Mount Pleasant Indian Industrial Boarding School." *International Journal of Historical Archaeology* 20 (3): 574–588.

Swan, Moses. 1874. *Ten Years and Ten Months in Lunatic Asylums in Different States.* Hoosick Falls: Printed for the author.

Swartz, Sally. 2005. "Can the Clinical Subject Speak?: Some Thoughts on Subaltern Psychology." *Theory & Psychology* 15 (4): 505–525.

Sweetser, William. 1850. *Mental Hygiene.* New York: George P. Putnam.

Tandberg, Ella to Rockwood Hoar. 11 July 1905. Rockwood Hoar Papers. Massachusetts Historical Society, Boston, Massachusetts.

Taylor, W. C. 1871. *A Physician's Counsels to Women, in Health and Disease.* Springfield: WJ Holland & Co.

Thomas, A. 1991. *Racism and Psychiatry.* Secaucus, NJ: Carol Publishing Group.

Thompson, Emily. 2002. *The Soundscape of Modernity.* Cambridge: MIT Press.

Thompson, Margaret S. 1985. "The Wages of Sin: The Problem of Alcoholism and General Paralysis in Nineteenth-Century Edinburgh." In *The Anatomy of Madness: Essays in the History of Psychiatry,* edited by W. F. Bynum and M. S. Shepherd, 316-336. London: Tavistock Publications.

Tilley, Christopher. 1994. *A Phenomenology of Landscape: Places, Paths, and Monuments.* Oxford: Berg.

Tomes, Nancy. 1984. *A Generous Confidence: Thomas Story Kirkbride and the Art of Asylum-Keeping, 1840-1883.* Cambridge: Cambridge University Press.

Topp, Leslie (2007). "The Modern Mental Hospital in Late 19th-Century Germany and Austria: Psychiatric Space and Images of Freedom and Control." In *Madness, Architecture, and the Built Environment: Psychiatric Spaces in Historical Context,* edited by Leslie Topp, James E. Moran, and Jonathan Andrews, 241–261. New York and London: Routledge.

Tromans, Nicholas. 2010. "The Psychiatric Sublime." Tate Papers No. 13. https://www.tate.org.uk/research/publications/tate-papers/13/the-psychiatric-sublime.

Tuke, Samuel. 1815. *Practical Hints on the Construction and Economy of Pauper Lunatic Asylums.* London: Printed for William Alexander.

Turner, Charles Henry to Harriet and Hattie Turner. 23 October 1877. Turner-Souther Family Papers, 1854–1912. Massachusetts Historical Society, Boston, MA.

Upshur, C. C., Paul R. Benson, Elizabeth Clemens, William H. Fisher, H. Stephen Leff, and Russell Schutt. 1997. "Closing State Mental Hospitals in Massachusetts: Policy, Process, and Impact." *International Journal of Law and Psychiatry* 20 (2): 199–217.

Van Deusen, E. H. 1869. *Observations on a Form of Nervous Prostration (Neurasthenia,) Culminating in Insanity.* Lansing: W. S. George & Co., Printers to the State.

Velez, A. 2018 "Effects of Soundscape on the Prairie Madness Phenomenon." 2018 Conference on Historical and Underwater Archaeology, New Orleans, LA, 3–6 January 2018.

Wall, Diana diZerega. 1994. *The Archaeology of Gender: Separating the Spheres in Urban America.* New York: Plenum Press.

Wetherbee, Jean. 1985. *A Second Look at White Ironstone.* Wallace Homestead Book Company.

White, M. J. 1893. "Adjuncts to Medical Treatment in Hospitals for the Insane." *American Journal of Insanity* 49 (4): 569–578.

White, M. J. 1893. "Adjuncts to Medical Treatment in Hospitals for the Insane." *American Journal of Insanity* 49 (4): 569–578.

Wigan, A. L. 1845. "A New View of Insanity: The Duality of the Mind Proved by the Structure, Functions, and Diseases of the Brain, and By the Phenomena of Mental Derangement, and Shown to Be Essential to Moral Responsibility." *American Journal of Insanity* 1 (4): 375–389.

Wilbur, H. B. to Pliny Earle. 29 January 1879. Pliny Earle Papers. American Antiquarian Society, Worcester, Massachusetts.

Willson, Mary to Lily Dana. 21 January 1889. Dana Family Papers. Massachusetts Historical Society, Boston, Massachusetts.

Woodward, Samuel B. [n.d.] "Medical Treatment of Insanity." Samuel B. Woodward Papers, American Antiquarian Society, Worcester, Mass.

Woodward, Samuel B. to Doctor Joseph Parish. 5 July 1845. Samuel B. Woodward Papers, American Antiquarian Society, Worcester, Mass.

Woodward, Samuel B. to his brother [unnamed]. 25 May 1831. Samuel B. Woodward Papers. American Antiquarian Society, Worcester, Massachusetts.

Woodward, Samuel B. to Horace Mann. 1 April 1833. Samuel B. Woodward Papers. American Antiquarian Society, Worcester, Massachusetts.

Woodward, Samuel B. to Horace Mann. 11 March 1832. Samuel B. Woodward Papers. American Antiquarian Society, Worcester, Massachusetts.

Wyman, Morrill. 1877. *The Early History of the McLean Asylum for the Insane: A Criticism of the Report of the Massachusetts State Board of Health for 1877.* Cambridge: Riverside Press.

Wynter, Rebecca 2010. "'Good in All Respects': Appearance and Dress at Staffordshire County Lunatic Asylum, 1818-54." *History of Psychiatry* 22 (1): 40–57.

Yanni, Carla. 2007. *The Architecture of Madness: Insane Asylums in the United States.* Minneapolis: University of Minnesota.

Index

agriculture. *See* farm

anthropology, 1, 22–26; medical. *See* medical anthropology; of the senses, 21–22, 25, 29

archaeology, 2, 21–27, 30, 176, 202; historical. *See* historical archaeology; of institutions, 22–23, 26–28, 176

architecture, 37–41, 44–45, 47–48, 51, 65, 110; Gothic Style, 37, 40, 47, 65; Neo-Palladian, 11, 93

Association of Medical Superintendents of American Institutions for the Insane (AMSAII), 41–42, 48, 89, 123, 133, 146, 193–94; 26 rules of, 41–42, 48

asylum literature, 11, 28, 81

attendants. *See* employees

Beers, Clifford, 7–8, 52, 58, 60, 83, 117–19, 123, 125, 126, 134, 140, 143, 166, 188, 190–91, 195, 199, 202, 204

Bell, Dr. Luther, 168–70

Bellevue Hospital, 60, 119

Bemis, Dr. Merrick, 90, 110, 160, 163

Blackwell's Island Asylum, 122, 142, 146, 181, 188, 193

Bloomingdale Insane Asylum, 111–13

Bly, Nelly, 8, 58, 60, 114–15, 118, 119, 181, 188, 193–94

Browne, Dr. W. A. F., 28, 37, 55, 89, 91, 97, 102, 113, 161, 167–69

capitalism, 3, 81, 136, 171, 184, 185, 199

ceramics, 22, 171–72, 176–81

chapel, 2, 30, 39, 79–80, 108, 116–18

clock tower, 27, 76, 77

clothing, 49, 53–58, 125

confinement, 8–9, 29–30, 38, 52, 65–66, 70, 84–88, 91–93, 101–2, 113, 119–20, 126–27, 150, 172, 188, 195, 202

Conolly, Dr. John, 98, 119–20, 141, 157, 160, 172

cottage plan, 90, 110, 154, 163

"cult of curability," 14, 17, 39, 47, 51, 53, 165

Danvers State Hospital, 89

deinstitutionalization, 20–21, 201–3

demolition, 26–27, 41

Denny, Lydia, 30, 85, 88, 102, 125, 190, 192–96

diet. *See* food

dining, 170–76, 184

discipline, 24, 35, 64, 97–98, 113, 121–22, 124–25, 147–48, 150, 157, 166, 171–72, 175–76, 184

Dix, Dorothea Lynde, 129, 145, 151–53, 196

domesticity, 52, 62–63, 69, 80–84, 100, 101, 175, 179, 180

Earle, Dr. Pliny, 15, 51–53, 78, 111–15, 120–21, 162, 171, 182
"Edifice Complex," 35, 47, 51
employees, 5, 13, 14, 19, 52, 55, 65, 100, 113, 116, 119–20, 122, 123, 126, 131, 135, 137, 138, 140–43, 146–48, 153–54, 172, 181–83, 189, 190, 194–95, 197, 200, 202
Esquirol, Etienne, 97, 144, 148, 149
expenditures, 48–49, 52–53, 84, 140, 180

farm, 19, 44–45, 162–66, 182, 203
farmhouse, 44, 163–64
fire, 26, 27, 40, 50–51, 132, 203
food, 155–85
forced feeding, 166–70
Foucault, Michel, 24–25, 82, 96–97, 102, 114, 150–51, 202
Freud, Dr. Sigmund, 115
Fuller, Robert, 8–9, 30, 64, 85, 91, 119, 188, 190, 192, 195, 196
furnishings, 56, 58–63, 77, 81–82, 84, 89, 102, 112–13, 149

gardens, 4, 11, 26, 41, 75, 82, 112, 201, 204
gender, 54, 77, 94–95, 179–80, 193–94, 199
Grob, Gerald, 15, 33, 142–43, 167, 198

Hanwell Asylum, 58, 120, 172
Hartford Retreat, 13, 30, 81
Haskell, Ebenezer, 8, 29, 33, 169, 188, 192
Hill, Elizabeth R., 85, 88, 91, 96, 118, 135, 143, 174
Hillside Farm, 44–46, 164
historical archaeology, 22–23, 27–28, 30
Hooper Turret and Gage Turret, 27, 77, 98–101
Hudson River State Hospital, 40
Hunt, Isaac, 8, 29, 194, 198, 199
hydrotherapy, 20, 131, 144–48, 194
hygiene, 32, 130–40, 143, 151–53, 198, 201
hysteria, 167

iatrogenesis, 8, 33, 88, 183, 191
immigrants, 44, 114–15, 141–43, 151, 160, 167, 183, 198
industrialization, 3, 4, 6, 17–18, 73–74, 103, 104, 124, 129–30, 156
insanity: causes of, 5–6, 148, 158, 168; curability of, 1, 14–17, 47, 114, 165; definition of, 5; as "disease of civilization," 1, 6, 156, 170, 173; medicalization of, 5–7
intersensoriality, 32, 187–90

Jacksonville Asylum, 9, 29, 44, 85, 88, 119, 122, 125, 174, 182, 189–91, 196
Jarvis, Dr. Edward, 17, 91, 116, 132, 136

Kirkbride, Dr. Thomas Story, 18, 28, 172, 194
Kirkbride plan, 18, 36, 40–41, 65, 77, 106

landscape, 18, 24, 27–28, 35, 37, 40, 70–77, 82, 101, 118
light, 11, 31, 71, 78–80, 82, 90–91, 116, 122, 134
location, 10–12, 71–76, 85, 105, 188
Locke, John, 6–7

Maine State Hospital, 8, 29, 199
Massachusetts: Board of State Charities, 89, 110; Department of Mental Health, 27, 202; State Commission of Lunacy, 17, 132–33; state legislature, 9–10; treatment of the insane in, 10, 17, 20, 57, 129, 132–33, 202, 204
materiality, 18, 22–28, 31, 35–41, 46, 48–49, 51–52, 60, 63, 65–66, 104, 114, 176
McLean Asylum, 11, 30, 64, 85, 91, 119, 122, 125, 137, 146, 162, 169, 173, 188, 190, 194–95
medical anthropology, 23–24
medicines, 121–23, 167; antipsychotic, 20, 146, 166; narcotic, 121–23, 158–59, 190
methodology, 26–31

Meyer, Dr. Adolf, 19, 51
Mitchell, Dr. S. Weir, 167
morality, 4, 53–54, 71, 82, 114, 116,
  142–43, 155, 158, 159, 164, 183
moral treatment, 3–4, 13, 35–38, 42, 46,
  57, 65–66, 78, 91, 96, 97, 100–101,
  104, 135–36, 142, 144, 148, 150,
  155, 160, 168, 172, 175–76, 184,
  195, 198, 202, 204
music, 2, 7, 81, 103–4, 115–18, 121, 189
Myerson, Dr. David J., 165

nature, 2, 4, 5, 37, 39, 45, 71, 103, 104,
  116, 136, 155–57, 159, 171, 184, 201
Nightingale, Florence, 79, 136–37
nonrestraint movement, 113, 122
Northampton State Hospital, 15, 17, 53,
  78, 113, 182
nurses: strike of, 19, 49, 120, 142, 182–
  83. *See also* employees

overcrowding, 2, 14, 15, 17, 19, 32, 36,
  42, 48, 108–10, 113, 118, 130, 132–
  37, 142, 151–52, 190, 194, 201

Packard, Elizabeth, 8–9, 44, 64, 85–86,
  88, 102, 119, 122, 125, 135, 140,
  143, 174, 181–82, 185, 189, 190,
  192–95, 199–200, 204
Panopticon, 98–100
patients: abuse of, 8, 9, 20, 86, 109, 110,
  119, 123, 141, 143–47, 194–96, 204;
  agency and protest of, 25, 36, 52–53,
  55–56, 62–64, 66, 70, 87–88, 101–2,
  110–11, 119, 124–26, 170, 184, 187–
  94, 198–200; belongings of, 58, 64;
  black, 14, 44, 151, 197; classification
  of, 11, 14, 36, 42, 51, 65, 106–9,
  161, 163–64, 174–75; deaths and
  burials of, 45–47, 66, 67, 85, 86, 123,
  168–69, 190; families of, 66, 80, 81,
  83, 84, 86–87, 89, 94, 123, 162, 195;
  female. *See* women; foreign-born.
  See immigrants; "incurable," 15–17,
  32, 44–46, 59, 83–84, 89, 102,

106–7, 159, 164–65, 173, 185, 191;
  Irish, 44, 142–43, 151, 160; labor by,
  2, 32, 93, 106–7, 121, 124, 137–38,
  161–66, 173, 180, 185, 199; pauper.
  See pauper lunatics; population of,
  16–17, 20, 26, 41–42, 66, 93, 107,
  109–10, 138, 140, 165–66, 174;
  portraits of, 94–97; private, 43, 60,
  65, 66, 81–82, 86, 137, 158–62, 173,
  176; suicidal, 27, 98–100; violent, 8,
  14, 36, 44, 53, 58–60, 82, 88, 101,
  109, 111, 118–19, 133, 134, 141,
  143, 152, 169, 184, 195
pauper lunatics, 14, 16–17, 22, 33, 43,
  46, 55, 65, 66, 70, 81, 86, 94, 129,
  158–61, 167, 173–74, 176, 183, 198
Pennsylvania Hospital, 8, 18, 29, 160,
  172, 188, 192
Pennsylvania System, 121–22
phenomenology, 2, 24
Pinel, Dr. Philippe, 13, 96, 144, 148, 172
plumbing, 42, 136–40, 152
prisons, 37, 44, 55, 65, 70, 81, 84–89,
  92, 97, 99, 101–2, 107, 122, 145,
  154, 190, 203

Quakers, 4, 13, 78, 122, 159

race, 44, 111, 149–52, 196–98
Ray, Dr. Isaac, 88, 100, 107, 148, 158
religion, 3–6, 16, 39, 78, 88, 122, 141,
  155–56, 169
restraint, 98, 100, 113, 120–22, 147–48,
  167–69
Romanticism, 37, 39, 71, 101, 104, 136,
  179
Royal Edinburgh Asylum, 125, 176, 180

sensorial assemblage, 2, 8, 25, 26, 30, 202
sight, 69–70, 93–97, 188, 189
slavery, 121, 152, 196–97
smell, 129–54, 188
social class, 3, 65, 69, 130, 136, 143,
  144, 151, 152, 157–62, 172–74, 176,
  183, 189, 198

social control, 21, 24, 26, 82, 99, 102, 148, 202
sound, 32, 83–84, 103–27, 189
Stone, Elizabeth, 30, 91, 122, 146, 188, 190–92, 194, 195
strong rooms, 38, 44, 52, 56, 70, 82, 84, 87–88, 106, 108–9, 133–35, 152, 174, 188–89, 198
Summer Street Department. *See* Worcester Asylum for the Chronic Insane
surveillance, 24, 27, 97–100
Swan, Moses, 8, 29, 64, 85–86, 109, 146, 190, 195, 199–200, 204

taste, 159, 166, 181. *See also* food
Taunton Lunatic Hospital, 29, 80, 87
tea parties, 170–76, 184
therapeutic pessimism, 15–16, 32, 135–36, 201
Titicut follies, 20
total institutions, 3, 150, 153
touch. *See* materiality
Troy Lunatic Asylum, 8, 29, 85, 109, 146, 190, 199, 204
Tuke, Samuel, 11, 28, 33, 90–91, 109
Turner, Charles Henry, 29, 80, 84, 87, 99

urbanization, 72–76, 78, 103–5, 129–30, 156–67
utopianism, 1, 4, 74, 97, 102, 113, 154

ventilation, 72, 90, 131–33, 149, 152
views, 39, 42, 71–78, 84, 91
viewshed analysis, 77–78

wards: furnishing of. *See* furnishings; segregation of, 14, 44, 46–47, 59, 70, 82, 85–87, 99–102, 106, 108–10, 115–16, 151, 176, 197; violent. *See* strong rooms
water supply, 137–40
Willard Asylum for the Chronic Insane, 43, 106, 165
windows, 11, 33, 38, 40–41, 61, 81, 84, 86, 88, 90–93, 131–34, 172, 188
women, 27, 56, 58, 77, 94–95, 98, 100, 117, 148–49, 151, 176, 179–80, 193–94, 197, 199
Woodward, Dr. Samuel B., 5–6, 13–14, 16, 39, 54, 59, 71–72, 81–82, 104, 116, 120, 142, 144, 145, 149, 160–62, 171–75, 183, 196, 198
Worcester Asylum for the Chronic Insane, 45
Worcester, city of, 10, 45, 71–72, 77, 139; growth of, 73–75, 105
Worcester Recovery Center and Hospital, 20, 203

York Retreat, 11, 13, 33, 90

About the Author

Madeline Kearin Ryan is a librarian and archivist at the Worcester Historical Museum and holds a PhD in archaeology from Brown University.

www.ingramcontent.com/pod-product-compliance
Lightning Source LLC
Chambersburg PA
CBHW050643280326
41932CB00015B/2766